EDUCATION IN A COMPETITIVE AND GLOBALIZING WORLD

EXPLORING THE OPPORTUNITIES AND CHALLENGES OF MEDICAL STUDENTS

EDUCATION IN A COMPETITIVE AND GLOBALIZING WORLD

Additional books and e-books in this series can be found on Nova's website under the Series tab.

EDUCATION IN A COMPETITIVE AND GLOBALIZING WORLD

EXPLORING THE OPPORTUNITIES AND CHALLENGES OF MEDICAL STUDENTS

ELIAS A. JESPERSEN
EDITOR

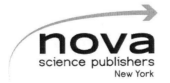

Copyright © 2019 by Nova Science Publishers, Inc.

All rights reserved. No part of this book may be reproduced, stored in a retrieval system or transmitted in any form or by any means: electronic, electrostatic, magnetic, tape, mechanical photocopying, recording or otherwise without the written permission of the Publisher.

We have partnered with Copyright Clearance Center to make it easy for you to obtain permissions to reuse content from this publication. Simply navigate to this publication's page on Nova's website and locate the "Get Permission" button below the title description. This button is linked directly to the title's permission page on copyright.com. Alternatively, you can visit copyright.com and search by title, ISBN, or ISSN.

For further questions about using the service on copyright.com, please contact:
Copyright Clearance Center
Phone: +1-(978) 750-8400   Fax: +1-(978) 750-4470   E-mail: info@copyright.com

NOTICE TO THE READER

The Publisher has taken reasonable care in the preparation of this book, but makes no expressed or implied warranty of any kind and assumes no responsibility for any errors or omissions. No liability is assumed for incidental or consequential damages in connection with or arising out of information contained in this book. The Publisher shall not be liable for any special, consequential, or exemplary damages resulting, in whole or in part, from the readers' use of, or reliance upon, this material. Any parts of this book based on government reports are so indicated and copyright is claimed for those parts to the extent applicable to compilations of such works.

Independent verification should be sought for any data, advice or recommendations contained in this book. In addition, no responsibility is assumed by the Publisher for any injury and/or damage to persons or property arising from any methods, products, instructions, ideas or otherwise contained in this publication.

This publication is designed to provide accurate and authoritative information with regard to the subject matter covered herein. It is sold with the clear understanding that the Publisher is not engaged in rendering legal or any other professional services. If legal or any other expert assistance is required, the services of a competent person should be sought. FROM A DECLARATION OF PARTICIPANTS JOINTLY ADOPTED BY A COMMITTEE OF THE AMERICAN BAR ASSOCIATION AND A COMMITTEE OF PUBLISHERS.

Additional color graphics may be available in the e-book version of this book.

Library of Congress Cataloging-in-Publication Data

ISBN: 978-1-53616-213-4

Published by Nova Science Publishers, Inc. † New York

Contents

Preface		vii
Chapter 1	Quality Improvement Education for Medical Students: A Systematic Review *Elizabeth Brooks, Anila Rao, Ashley Harnden, Lori Mills, Thomas Alderson, James McQuiston and Grace D. Brannan*	1
Chapter 2	Experiential Research and Scholarly Programs for Medical Students: Short-Term Paradigms *Clarissa Dass, Melissa Ianitelli, David Tolentino, Jody Gerome, Nicole Wadsworth and Grace D. Brannan*	31
Chapter 3	Leadership Development Programs in Undergraduate Medical Education: Understanding the Need, Best Practices and Challenges *Sumita Sethi*	57

Chapter 4	Comparison of Idealistic Commitments between First and Third Year Medical Students *Sabrina F. Merino, Lorena E. López Balbuena, Ana María Rancich, Ricardo J. Gelpi and Martín Donato*	**89**
Chapter 5	Can Code Switching Complement Learning? Saudi Arabian Medical Students' Perceptions of English as the Language of Instruction *Mohammed Alenezi and Paul Kebble*	**105**
Chapter 6	Social Skills of Physicians and Medical Students: Problem Overview (from Experience of Ukraine) *Lesya V. Lymar*	**129**
Index		**151**
Related Nova Publications		**155**

PREFACE

Exploring the Opportunities and Challenges of Medical Students begins with a systematic review of quality improvement curricula for medical students to identify current training techniques, learning outcomes, opportunities, and challenges to the implementation of quality improvement curricula.

Following this, the authors describe the curricula and analyze results from two short term programs: a summer research and scholarly program between the first and second year of medical school, and research rotation electives offered to third- and fourth- year students.

The authors also discuss the rationale for developing physician-leaders, review the need for incorporating leadership development programs in medical curriculum, and discuss the best practices of formulating such programs and their expected challenges.

This compilation goes on to compare first and third year medical students' commitments in relation to idealism, as several works have demonstrated that idealism decreases as the students' progress in their career, partially due to the hidden curriculum.

Using questionnaires as data collection instruments, one included paper reports on the qualitative analysis of responses and subsequent discussion in English, including implications and recommendations for Saudi Arabian medical education authorities to better achieve the objectives of medical education through the medium of language instruction.

Lastly, this collection describes the notion of physicians' social skills (with emphasis on shaping social skills in medical students during their studies) in Ukraine, a country in which health services have undergone difficult changes after 1991.

Chapter 1 - To perform a systematic review of quality improvement (QI) curricula for medical students to identify current training techniques, learning outcomes, opportunities, and challenges to implementing QI curricula. Publications in PUBMED, SCOPUS, and EMBASE from January 1, 2009 to December 31, 2018 were identified using a structured search strategy in accordance with the PRISMA (Preferred Reporting Items for Systematic Reviews and Meta-Analyses) guidelines. A total of 29 studies with QI training or interventions involving medical students were identified. Themes regarding curricula implementation were identified across the articles. Most medical students involved in QI programs demonstrated improvement in QI knowledge and satisfaction with the experience. QI initiatives were seen across all years of medical education with a variety of educational delivery methods. Relative to previous systematic reviews on quality improvement with medical students, there is an increase in studies that describe organizational level changes (69.0%, n=20) and patient benefit (27.6%, n=8).

Factors including lack of clear curricular structure, interest, and time constraints decreased the effectiveness of curricular implementation. Successful quality improvement initiatives may require a multimodal curriculum with strong faculty support that occurs throughout preclinical and clinical years of medical school.

Chapter 2 - The decline in physician scientists has prompted attention from the medical field. With increasing focus on evidence-based medicine, there is an ongoing need to enhance research education for medical trainees. The undergraduate medical profession has recognized the need with the development of Entrustable Professional Activity or EPA by the Association of American Medical Colleges. Specifically, EPA 7 speaks to evidence-based medicine which is rooted in research and scholarly skills. This puts additional emphasis on research during medical school. To further highlight the importance of research, The Accreditation Council for Graduate Medical Education, the accrediting body for residency, requires that residents participate in research and scholarly activities. As such, it is very critical that medical students are equipped with research skills and experience to effectively meet residency requirements. Where schools may be challenged is providing experiential or hands-on opportunities. Some schools have added a fifth year to include research projects as a critical component. Dual degrees such as an MD/PhD and DO/PhD are also common. However, not all medical students will have the opportunity or interest to engage in these long-term programs. The objective of this chapter was to describe the curricula and analyze results from two short term programs: a Summer Research and Scholarly Program between the first and second year of medical school and Research Rotation Electives offered to third- and fourth-year students.

This chapter describes an IRB-approved study which involved a retrospective review of data accumulated over several years. Descriptive data was generated and analyzed. Student participation in both programs increased over the years. Students were statistically significantly ($p=0.00001$) mentored by more physicians compared to research scientists. There were subsequently significantly more students in both programs involved in clinical studies ($p=0.00001$). Participation by gender was not significantly different for summer ($p=0.372$) or elective participants ($p=0.105$). Summer researchers were mostly involved in data collection while elective students were increasingly involved in other activities such as proposal development and also took on more responsibility ($p=0.00001$). The increase noted in both programs and the equal participation of female and male medical students were very encouraging. The authors also described the curricula to provide detail to readers who are creating their own curriculum on short-term programs to provide hands-on research opportunities for students.

Chapter 3 - The decline in physician scientists has prompted attention from the medical field. With increasing focus on evidence-based medicine, there is an ongoing need to enhance research education for medical trainees. The undergraduate medical profession has recognized the need with the development of Entrustable Professional Activity or EPA by the Association of American Medical Colleges. Specifically, EPA 7 speaks to evidence-based medicine which is rooted in research and scholarly skills. This puts additional emphasis on research during medical school. To further highlight the importance of research, The Accreditation Council for Graduate Medical Education, the accrediting body for residency, requires that residents participate in research and scholarly activities. As such, it is very critical that medical students are equipped with research skills and experience to effectively meet residency requirements. Where schools may be challenged is providing experiential or hands-on opportunities. Some schools have added a fifth year to include research projects as a critical component. Dual degrees such as an MD/PhD and DO/PhD are also common. However, not all medical students will have the opportunity or interest to engage in these long-term programs. The objective of this chapter was to describe the curricula and analyze results from two short term programs: a Summer Research and Scholarly Program between the first and second year of medical school and Research Rotation Electives offered to third- and fourth-year students.

This chapter describes an IRB-approved study which involved a retrospective review of data accumulated over several years. Descriptive data was generated and analyzed. Student participation in both programs increased over the years. Students were statistically significantly ($p=0.00001$) mentored by more physicians compared to research scientists. There were subsequently significantly more students in both programs involved in clinical studies ($p=0.00001$). Participation by gender was not significantly different for summer ($p=0.372$) or elective participants ($p=0.105$). Summer researchers were mostly involved in data collection while elective students were increasingly involved in other activities such as proposal development and also took on more responsibility ($p=0.00001$). The increase noted in both programs and the equal participation of female and male medical students were very encouraging. The authors also described the curricula to provide detail to readers who are creating their own curriculum on short-term programs to provide hands-on research opportunities for students.

Chapter 4 - *Introduction:* Medicine is a career that could attract students with humanistic ideals. Idealism in medicine is understood as the pursuit of improved quality of life and relief of suffering for humankind, with emphasis on underserved populations. Several works have demonstrated that idealism decreases as the students' progress in their career, partially due to the hidden curriculum. The aim of this study is to compare first and third year medical students' commitments in relation to idealism and analyze their differences.

Material and methods: The authors administered an anonymous and voluntary survey to first and third year medical students of an Argentine university. The students had to answer demographic questions first and then write a maximum of 7 ethical compromises they would like to commit to as graduates. Only those commitments related to idealism were selected. The analysis between the variables was performed with the chi square test (P<0,05).

Results: A total of 1497 ethical commitments were obtained in first year and 1402 in third year. Out of those, 263 (17.6%) and 118 (8.4%) commitments, in first and third year respectively, were related to idealism. They referred to: the principle of justice and working with underserved populations; be a committed physician doing more than required; not use the medical profession as means for profit; follow ethics and morals and be an example for others; improve public health; be loyal to one's beliefs; obey the law and fight for human rights; save lives. The formulation of these commitments decrease in third year, being the relation between the variables was statistically significant ($X^2 = 27.47$; $P = 0.0003$).

Discussion: The authors' results show a decrease in the formulation of idealistic commitments in third year that could be attributed to the hidden curriculum. Possible explanations could be the increased exposure to the medical profession, through the exchange of stories and anecdotes with professors and peers. Having taken the subject Bioethics and learning about

Principialism with emphasis in patient's autonomy could have led third year students to express commitments more related to the doctor-patient relationship in particular and less with society in general. Also, the study of biomedical sciences and the lack of humanistic disciplines (only Bioethics and Mental Health during the first three years) would create a more technical mindset in the students, leaving aside issues related to the medical responsibility towards society.

Conclusion: The authors' study suggests that there is a decline in students' idealism in the first three years of medical school possibly due to the hidden curriculum.

Chapter 5 - English language plays a crucial role in the delivery of medical education globally due to the vast body of medical related resources available only in English. This is clearly visible with most colleges and universities around the world offering medical and health science courses exclusively in English. Simultaneously textbooks and reference learning materials for medical education are available only in English. To benefit from this linguistic trend, Saudi Arabian education authorities have incorporated English as the language of instruction for medical education in the Kingdom. To meet the learning and teaching requirements, along with Saudi Arabian academics teaching faculty in the Kingdom's medical colleges have been recruited from a variety of countries including USA, UK, South Africa, India, Egypt, Sudan, Syria and Pakistan. With English being the supposed sole medium of instruction within the classrooms, the linguistic expectations of these recruits is a proven high level of competency in English. The faculty members from Saudi Arabia and from other Arab countries, however, often prefer to mix English and Arabic in their linguistic medium of instruction and interaction in their teaching. From a learner's perspective, it requires noting that English, being a foreign language in the Kingdom of Saudi Arabia, poses diverse challenges to Saudi medical students. As a language of instruction and interaction inside the classroom, the switching between English and Arabic receives mixed reactions from both instructors and students. The engaged code-switching (English-Arabic/Arabic-English) is perceived to be beneficial by some, while others view it as a substantial obstacle in mastering the target language, English. This blended, interwoven linguistic relationship between English and Arabic inside some Saudi Arabian medical classrooms, along with the perceptions of teachers and students towards the same, are explored in the current paper. Using questionnaires as data collection instruments, the paper reports on the qualitative analysis of responses and subsequent discussion. This includes direct implications and consequential recommendations for Saudi Arabian medical education authorities to better achieve the objectives of medical education through the medium of English language instruction in the Kingdom of Saudi Arabia.

Chapter 6 - The chapter describes the notion of the physician's social skills and their structure, with emphasis on shaping social skills in medical students during their medical studies. The paper deals with the peculiarities of medical social skills in Ukraine as a country the Health Service of which has undergone rather difficult changes after 1991. Social skills of a physician represent his knowledge, abilities and skills of productive interpersonal interaction with the patient, according to the standards accepted in the society and medical environment, which benefit both sides; good social skills are essential for a well-performing physician. It is a rare case when the person enters Medical School with the already well-shaped social skills; social skills of a medical student usually need correction, in Ukraine particularly.

The following components within the structure of the physician's social skills have been defined: motivation, cognition, emotions, management and communication. Predominance of professional motives, combined with scientific and social motives, compose the efficient social skills' motivation component. The cognition component of social skills of the physician is represented with the physician's knowledge on the essence, factors and strategies of productive interaction with others. The management component of the physician's social skills is represented with various behavior practical abilities and skills of productive interaction, well-developed skills of self-analysis, etc. The emotional component of social skills, represented with the average "moderate" empathy expression, will provide for t productive interaction and prevention of conflicts. The communication component of social skills is represented with the physician's tendency to perceive the patient as an equal communication partner. All these components should be closely monitored in medical students and corrected throughout their medical studies, before they start their practice with the patients, using the methods described in the chapter.

In: Exploring the Opportunities ...
Editor: Elias A. Jespersen

ISBN: 978-1-53616-213-4
© 2019 Nova Science Publishers, Inc.

Chapter 1

QUALITY IMPROVEMENT EDUCATION FOR MEDICAL STUDENTS: A SYSTEMATIC REVIEW

Elizabeth Brooks[1,5], DO, Anila Rao[1,5], DO, Ashley Harnden[2,5], DO, Lori Mills[3,5], Thomas Alderson[4,5], DO, James McQuiston[2,5], DO and Grace D. Brannan[6,*], PhD

[1]Department of Internal Medicine,
[2]Department of General Surgery,
[3]Department of Graduate Medical Education,
[4]Department of Obstetrics and Gynecology,
[5]College of Osteopathic Medicine,
Michigan State University, East Lansing, MI, US
[6]GDB Research and Statistical Consulting, Athens, OH, US

---

* Corresponding Author's Email: gracebrannan2013@gmail.com.

Abstract

To perform a systematic review of quality improvement (QI) curricula for medical students to identify current training techniques, learning outcomes, opportunities, and challenges to implementing QI curricula. Publications in PUBMED, SCOPUS, and EMBASE from January 1, 2009 to December 31, 2018 were identified using a structured search strategy in accordance with the PRISMA (Preferred Reporting Items for Systematic Reviews and Meta-Analyses) guidelines. A total of 29 studies with QI training or interventions involving medical students were identified. Themes regarding curricula implementation were identified across the articles. Most medical students involved in QI programs demonstrated improvement in QI knowledge and satisfaction with the experience. QI initiatives were seen across all years of medical education with a variety of educational delivery methods. Relative to previous systematic reviews on quality improvement with medical students, there is an increase in studies that describe organizational level changes (69.0%, n=20) and patient benefit (27.6%, n=8).

Factors including lack of clear curricular structure, interest, and time constraints decreased the effectiveness of curricular implementation. Successful quality improvement initiatives may require a multimodal curriculum with strong faculty support that occurs throughout preclinical and clinical years of medical school.

Keywords: quality improvement training and education, undergraduate medical students, curriculum

1. Introduction

The publication of the Institute of Medicine's report, *Crossing the Quality Chasm*, in 2001 shined a light on the broken American healthcare system and the need for quality improvement (QI) [1]. The Institute of Medicine released their landmark report *To Err is Human: Building a Safer Health System* demonstrating tens of thousands of patients die each year in the hospital as a result of medical error [2]. What was once taken for granted as common sense or "good practice" has now turned into specific guidelines and core competencies for medical students and residents alike to combat these concerns. Over the last decade, medical education has witnessed a transformation in QI and patient safety (PS) concerns. The Association of American Medical Colleges (AAMC) Core Entrustable Professional Activities for Entering Residency regards a trainee's ability to analyze their environment and performance as a physician using quality improvement methods as a critical competency [3].

Despite recognizing QI skills as a necessary competency, the AAMC found many graduating medical students in 2010 did not believe they received enough instruction on QI [4, 5]. In a survey of third year medical students, 57.1% had not been exposed to QI and 82.6% had not been exposed to Plan, Do, Study, Act (PDSA) [6]. Moreover, at least 60% of these students thought that QI was as important as the basic science and clinical curricula.

In order to foster QI skills, South African medical schools began to incorporate education and application of QI in their curriculum [4]. In sub-Saharan African medical schools, at least 45% (5/11) were teaching at least one of the aspects of quality of care to their medical students during the six-year program [7]. Approximately 80% of these schools (4/5) educated their students about error reporting and handling.

Medical education organizations have also been actively promoting QI. The Association of American Medical Colleges' (AAMC) Aligning and Educating Quality initiative promotes medical schools to develop programs that encourage education about quality improvement at the earliest stages of medical careers [8]. In addition, AAMC's Entrustable Professional Activity outlines 13 activities that a medical student must be able to execute at the beginning of residency [3]. QI is one of the required activities. QI's importance is further emphasized in residency by the Accreditation Council for Graduate Medical Education (ACGME) where it is part of the Common Program Requirements that residents need to meet [9]. QI is also a critical component of ACGME's Clinical Learning Environment Review for residencies [10].

QI projects can potentially impact medical students' opportunities to transform healthcare. In a qualitative study by Bergh et al. [11], QI projects were part of a health rotation curriculum. In addition to completing the projects which helped the clinical site, students were able to demonstrate growth in critical thinking and team dynamics.

A few comprehensive reviews have been completed in the past few years that informed this chapter. Wong et al. in 2010 performed a systematic review of quality improvement and patient safety training of both medical students and residents [12]. Most of the studies that met the authors' criteria were focused on residents. Common QI topics taught were continuous QI, systems thinking, and root cause analysis. Improved knowledge was observed in most curricula and 32% resulted in a change in the delivery of care and 17% resulted in improvement. Kirkman et al. followed in 2015 with a systematic review for both residents and medical students but focused only on patient safety [13]. Some QI concepts such as root cause analysis and systems-based analysis were included in the curricula, but the application was specific to patient safety. Jones et al. in 2015 conducted a realist review of QI/PS studies involving both students and residents but limited to the clinical setting and included articles from 2000 to 2013 [14]. The study's focus was to determine the effects of teaching QI in the clinical setting to improve knowledge, patient care, and system performance. They found that factors such as trained faculty and choice of project for trainees contributed to a successful clinical QI curriculum. Kirkman and Jones' studies were focused solely on patient safety or QI in the clinical setting in both medical students and residents, respectively [13, 14]. All three studies involved both residents and medical students. What was evident was a need for a comprehensive review of QI training and curriculum focused specifically on medical students.

Our goal in this chapter was to perform a systematic review from January 1, 2009 to December 31, 2018 to determine the current training and curriculum opportunities as well as challenges faced specifically in teaching quality improvement to medical students. Reviewing the current state of medical student education relating to these measures will allow educators to see best practices and where further work needs to be done. Focusing on medical students allows for QI training at the fundamental and formative level, prior to trainees' exposure to patients and hospitals, which could lead to a focus on preventative medicine while cultivating an improvement mindset.

2. METHODS

2.1. Literature Search

We established a search strategy consistent with the PRISMA (Preferred Reporting Items for Systematic reviews and Meta-Analyses) guidelines. We utilized the electronic databases PUBMED, SCOPUS, and EMBASE with a search period from January 1, 2009 to December 31, 2018. The purpose of this search period was to effectively find articles that have been published since the last relevant systematic review covering this topic [12]. The search was last conducted on March 15, 2019.

The search strategies focused primarily on quality improvement in medical education. We identified synonyms for "medical education," "quality improvement," and "curriculum" based on Medical Subject Heading (MeSH) terms and key terms identified in relevant articles. The three main ideas were combined using the Boolean operator "and" while synonyms were combined using "or." The detailed PUBMED search strategy is in Appendix 1. We did not limit our search to "human" studies only as we found too many studies were not indexed by this filter. Only articles published in the English language were considered, and all duplicate articles were removed among the databases.

2.2. Eligibility Criteria

We included articles on QI training or curriculum involving medical students. Any articles that involved other healthcare trainees (i.e., nursing students or residents) were included as long as medical students were involved. We defined an educational intervention to include one or more of the following as core contents: human factors, systems thinking, or root cause analysis. We determined several identifying terms related to QI and included articles which involved one of these concepts (i.e., quality improvement, systems-based practice, process mapping, root cause analysis, PDSA, incident reporting, error disclosure, patient safety). Articles discussing patient safety were only included if the intervention was taught alongside QI. Studies were excluded if they were a systematic review or meta-analysis, commentary, letter, or editorial.

2.3. Article Review Process

A medical librarian (LM) identified a total of 3,889 articles by our search strategies. After duplicates were removed, titles and abstracts were reviewed by four physicians in teams of two (TA and EB; AH and JM) using a double screening process in Abstrackr (Brown University, Providence, RI). Disagreements were reviewed by an additional researcher (GB). All abstracts meeting inclusion criteria were also double screened through a full article review by all researchers. A total of 29 articles were determined to meet the full inclusion criteria [4, 8, 15-41].

For comparison, we identified fundamental components in each article including study population, intervention performed, educational QI component, major findings, and learning outcomes. We utilized the Kirkpatrick's model to determine the trainee learning outcomes: impact on learners' satisfaction, changes in attitudes, knowledge and skills, changes in learners' behavior, organizational changes, and patient benefits [42]. Simple descriptive statistics such as frequency and percentage were generated to summarize the results.

3. RESULTS

3.1. Selected Articles

Our initial screening criteria resulted in 3,889 citations identified in our search of PUBMED (931), EMBASE (1,417) and SCOPUS (1,541). Figure 1 shows the schematic diagram for the selection process. There were 1,485 duplicate articles removed leaving us with 2,404 abstracts that were reviewed. Each article was randomly double screened to ensure optimal inclusion. During the review process 1,793 articles (74.6%) were excluded by title alone, whereas 513 articles (21.3%) were excluded by abstract; consensus amongst reviewers was to default to abstract exclusion if it was in any way unclear by title alone to avoid excluding potentially relevant articles. There were 98 articles obtained for full review. Our criteria of inclusion were articles that involved quality improvement education with direct curricular implementation on medical students. Articles with other health-care providers or trainees (e.g., registered nurses (RNs), residents, attendings, etc.) were also included as long as medical students were directly studied as well. To investigate a new area and differentiate this chapter from previous reviews, studies that solely looked at patient safety without quality improvement were excluded. Ultimately 29 final articles met our full inclusion criteria in our review (Table 1).

3.2. Characteristics of Studies

Among the 29 articles included, 23 articles were from the United States of America (USA) (79.3%) and 6 were international (20.7%); 2 in the United Kingdom, 1 in South Africa, 1 in Australia, 1 in New Zealand, and 1 in Canada (Table 2). A total of 26 (89.7%) articles were single institution studies and 3 were multi-institution studies (10.3%). Pre- and post-test and cohort designs comprised the majority of studies included. About 24% were qualitative (17.2%) or mixed methods (6.9%).

Sample size varied amongst the studies. Medical students alone were involved in 21 studies (72.4%), whereas 8 articles included medical students with other healthcare members (27.6%). Specifically, other healthcare members included in these 8 articles were nursing students, Masters students in health administration, respiratory therapy students, physician assistants, medical residents, faculty attending physicians or faculty from other academic programs (nursing, public health, allied healthy, dentistry and pharmacy). Seven studies specifically involved medical students in the pre-clinical years (1st and 2nd) (24.1%), 11 studies involved clinical year medical students (3rd and 4th) (37.9%), and 11 studies were a mixture of pre-clinical and clinical year medical students or unspecified (37.9%).

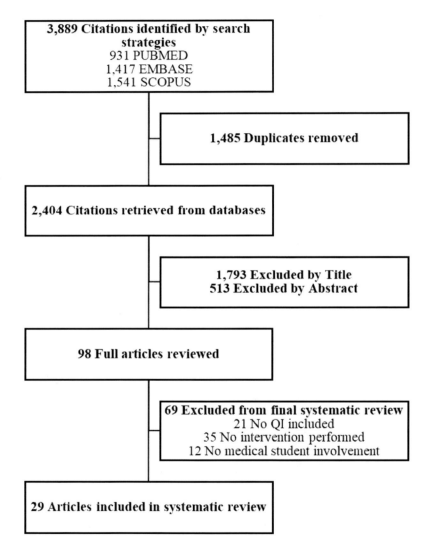

Figure 1. Schematic diagram showing the abstract and article selection process.

Table 1. Summary of 29 articles included in the study

First Author and Year / Country of Origin / Number of Primary Institution/s	Participants	Study Design/Teaching methods	Kirkpatrick's Level of Evaluation/Educational QI Content	Major Findings
Bac, 2015 [4] / South Africa/ Single	139 MS in final 18 months of program	Qualitative study/Project, small groups	1, 3, 4a, 4b/Plan Do Study Act (PDSA), Audit	Longitudinal QI projects can be successfully incorporated in an obstetrics rotation and resulted in hospital baby-friendly re-accreditation.
Manning, 2017 [8] / USA / Multiple	264 MS3 evaluated by 44 emergency physicians	Cohort/Project	4a, 4b/Literature search, A3 problem solving, PDSA, process flow, fishbone diagram, Lean, stakeholder assessment, Root cause analysis (RCA)	84% of physicians felt the students were effective, 86% were comfortable with students being a part of future QI initiatives.
Bartlett, 2018 [15] / USA / Single	22 MS1-4	Pre- and post-test/Extracurricular, project, Institute of Healthcare Improvement Open School (IHIOS), lecture, group sessions	1, 2b, 3, 4a, 4b/Basic QI, PDSA, RCA	Projects decreased *C. difficile* test orders. Knowledge score significantly increase (p<.01).
Bradham, 2018 [16] / USA / Single	132 MS3-4	Cohort/IHIOS, lectures, QI project	2a, 3, 4a/Fishbone diagram, process flow, 5 whys, key stakeholder assessment	132 students completed resulting in 110 completed QI projects; 70% rated its clinical relevance highly.

Table 1. (Continued)

First Author and Year / Country of Origin / Number of Primary Institution/s	Participants	Study Design/Teaching methods	Kirkpatrick's Level of Evaluation/Educational QI Content	Major Findings
Brown, 2018 [17] / Canada / Single	200 MS1 (83-in 2018 and 117 in 2019)	Mixed methods/Lecture; Used education as a case study	2a, 2b, 3, 4a/PDSA; basic QI	Lead to increase in QI knowledge.
Burnett, 2018 [18] / UK / Single	8 MS2 and MS3, 6- MS5s, 2 academic mentors and 5 clinical mentors	Qualitative study/IHIOS and project	4a, 4b/Human factors, systems engineering	QI projects in the clinical setting can teach skills but completion can be affected by time and roles and responsibilities between staff and students.
Chen, 2014 [19] / USA / Single	228 MS1-4	Pre- and post-test/Project	4a, 4b/Literature search, PDSA	A student clinic was a means to teach QI to students; project resulted in a decrease in patient visit time.
Cox, 2009 [20] / USA / Single	440 MS2, 250 nursing, 80 Masters in health administration, and 17 junior respiratory therapy students	Pre- and post-test/Lecture, simulation/cases, small groups	2a, 2b/Literature search, RCA, Failure Mode and Effects Analysis (FMEA), gap analysis, basic QI, process flow	Medical students were less likely than nursing students to believe that punishment should follow error.
Dumenco, 2018 [21] / USA / Single	136 MS1	Pre- and post-test/Mandatory, lecture, IHIOS, small groups	1, 2b/PDSA, RCA, fishbone diagram	Significant growth from pretest (65%) to posttest (89%); overall satisfaction over a 2-year period was 75% (i.e., good to very good).

First Author and Year / Country of Origin / Number of Primary Institution/s	Participants	Study Design/Teaching methods	Kirkpatrick's Level of Evaluation/Educational QI Content	Major Findings
Dysinger, 2011 [22] / USA / Single	510 MS4	Qualitative study/Project embedded in a required rotation; small group	1, 4a/PDSA	510 completed; 53% rated projects as "excellent"/"above average."
Elghouche, 2016 [23] / USA/ Single	29-6 medical students applying to otolaryngology, 7 otolaryngology and 7 psychiatry residents, and 9 faculty and staff	Cohort/Lecture, project	1, 3, 4a/Lean	29 (6 MS) completed the Yellow Lean Belt curriculum.
Hall, 2009 [24] / USA / Single	86 learners- 30 MS4, 56 allied professions	Cohort/Small groups, QI project	2b, 4a, 4b/PDSA, process flow, RCA, key stakeholder assessment	Experiential process facilitated QI skills and increased knowledge.
Huntington, 2009 [25] / USA / Multiple	16-10 MS and 6 nursing	Nonrandomized, Controlled Trial/Voluntary, Workbook-based, project	1, 2a, 2b, 4a/Basic QI	Test group had higher self-efficacy and confidently disseminated their findings via formal poster presentation.
Jackson, 2018 [26] / UK / Single	273 MS4	Qualitative Study/Audit or PDSA project	3, 4a/PDSA, Audit	QI experience was perceived as valuable by students. Audit was still preferred over PDSA because of time constraints.
James, 2016 [27] / USA / Single	230 students MS3	Cohort/Lecture, IHIOS, small groups, simulation	1, 2a, 2b, 3/System-based approach, RCA, basic QI, PDSA	Program was perceived as valuable and is now an interprofessional activity with nursing and pharmacy students.

Table 1. (Continued)

First Author and Year / Country of Origin / Number of Primary Institution/s	Participants	Study Design/Teaching methods	Kirkpatrick's Level of Evaluation/Educational QI Content	Major Findings
Kool, 2017 [28] / New Zealand / Single	32 MS6 (participated in evaluation), administrators, and staff	Mixed Methods/Lecture, project within obstetrics rotation	1, 2a, 2b, 4a/Literature search, audit	There is agreement among students (91%), clinicians (85%) and hospital QI and data management staff (70%) that the project gave students useful insights into QI in obstetrics.
Kutaimy, 2018 [29] / USA / Single	308 MS1	Pre- and post-test/Lecture, IHIOS, Simulation integrated into an anatomy lab	2a, 2b, 3/basic QI	Mean knowledge improved from 7.58 to 8.98 (p=0.000). Mean attitudes score improved from 47.73 to 50.56 (p=0.000).
Levitt, 2012 [30] / USA / Single	8 MS3	Pre- and post-test/Lecture, QI project	1, 2a, 2b/PDSA, key stakeholder assessment, RCA	Attitude improved from pre-test (9.9) vs post-test (12.6) (p=0.03). One of a few challenges were that proposals lacked enough analysis.
Margalit, 2009 [31] / USA / Single	155 students (34 MS) and 30 faculty from 6 medical and allied health programs	Pre- and post-test/Voluntary, lectures and small group	1, 2a, 2b/System error and practice, patient satisfaction	Improved awareness of health care quality and interprofessional teamwork principles.
Mauldon, 2014 [32] / Australia / Single	29 physician and staff evaluated 46 MS4	Qualitative study/Lecture and audit of diabetes care	4a, 4b/Audit	Learned clinical audit and contributed to the robustness of patient records at their site.

First Author and Year / Country of Origin / Number of Primary Institution/s	Participants	Study Design/Teaching methods	Kirkpatrick's Level of Evaluation/Educational QI Content	Major Findings
Miller, 2014 [33] / USA / Single	110 MS1 and allied health students	Pre- and post-test/IHIOS courses, small groups	2b/Basic QI	Significant differences in 16 of 16 and 13 of 16 (p=0.05) IHIOS courses for MS1 and allied health students, respectively.
Miller, 2015 [34] / USA / Multiple	601 MS1 and MS3 allied health students from 8 schools and 13 health disciplines	Cohort/IHIOS, small groups	2b/Basic QI	Significant learning was seen in all students (p=0.05). Successfully used the IHIOS chapters for interprofessional training delivery.
Mookherjee, 2013 [35] / USA / Single	6 MS4	Pre- and post-test/IHIOS, didactics, QI proposal	2a, 2b, 4a/PDSA	Improvement was observed but was not statistically significant.
Ogrinc, 2011 [36] / USA / Single	Approximately 440 MS2 students over 4 years	Cohort/Elective, Lecture and project	4a/PDSA, process flow diagram, RCA	Over 4 years, 22 (5% of class/year) completed 9 projects that impacted local level changes at a hospital.
O'Neill, 2013 [37] / USA / Single	197 MS1-4	Pre- and post-test/Project	2a, 2b, 3, 4a/Audit	Perceived QI skills significantly increased for all metrics in a longitudinal clerkship structure.
Paxton, 2010 [38] / USA / Single	40 MS3 (Medical Student), 6 MS4, and 5 Physician Assistant students; (35 completed a long-term posttest)	Pre- and post-test/Lecture, small groups	2b/RCA; Human factors analysis	Correct scores increased from pre-test (29.3%) to post-test (73.7%) (p<.001).

Table 1. (Continued)

First Author and Year / Country of Origin / Number of Primary Institution/s	Participants	Study Design/Teaching methods	Kirkpatrick's Level of Evaluation/Educational QI Content	Major Findings
Sweigart, 2016 [39] / USA / Single	6 MS2 from 4 institutions	Pre- and post-test/Lecture, shadowing, project	1, 2a, 2b, 3, 4a, 4b/Process mapping, RCA, PDSA	Average cumulative QIKAT results improved significantly (8.33 to 9.83, p=.04). Students continued other QI work beyond program.
Tartaglia, 2015 [40] / USA / Single	22 MS4-intervention and 12 MS4-control	Control vs Interventional/ IHIOS, mentored QI project	1, 2a, 2b, 4a/PDSA	QI curriculum demonstrated increased QI comfort and knowledge between test and control groups (p<0.05).
Vinci, 2014 [41] / USA / Single	23 MS1-4	Pre- and post-test/IHIOS, project	2a, 2b, 4a/Basic QI	Comfort and core QI skills improved.

Table 2. Study characteristics

Factors		Number of Studies	Percentage of All Studies (n=29)
Study Origin	USA	23	79.3%
	International	6	20.7%
Study Design	Controlled trials	2	6.9%
	Pre- and post- test	13	44.8%
	Cohort	7	24.1%
	Qualitative	5	17.2%
	Mixed methods	2	6.9%
Number of Institutions Involved	Single institution	26	89.7%
	Multiple institutions	3	10.3%
Participants	Medical students only	21	72.4%
	Medical students with others (Allied Health, Residents, Faculty, etc.)	8	27.6%

3.3. Kirkpatrick's Level of Evaluation

In the 29 studies reviewed we assessed the levels of evaluation using the Kirkpatrick's Model. All five of the different levels were represented in the studies in a variety of combinations (Table 3). Level 2b: Modification of knowledge/skill (65.5%) and Level 4a: Change in organizational practice (69%) were found to be most prevalent across the studies. Focus group discussions, questionnaires, surveys, interviews, and pre and post tests were used to determine the students' assessments of the QI training and experiences.

Table 3. Kirkpatrick's levels of evaluation

Level of Evaluation	Number of Studies	Percentage of All Studies (n=29)
Level 1: Participation	12	41.4%
Level 2a: Modification of attitudes/perceptions	14	48.3%
Level 2b: Modification of knowledge/skills	19	65.5%
Level 3: Behavioral change	10	34.5%
Level 4a: Change in organizational practice	20	69.0%
Level 4b: Benefits to patients	8	27.6%

3.4. Curriculum Content and Evaluation

The curricular features were expectedly varied with many teaching methods used. Curricula were mainly evaluated by students only (55.2%) followed by evaluation by both staff and students (31.0%). For the remaining studies, evaluations were completed by staff only (13.8%).

The majority of studies (n=17; 58.6%) did involve classic learning through lectures and didactics. There were 20 studies (69.0%) which involved a project. The use of the Institute for Healthcare Improvement Open School (IHIOS) online modules was high at 37.9% or in 11 studies.

Various QI approaches and tools were used in the different studies. Predominantly, most curricula included PDSA (51.7%) followed by root cause analysis (34.5%) and basic QI principles and tools (31.0%). QI was predominantly taught as a mandatory rotation or embedded in a mandatory rotation/curriculum (51.7%).

Table 4. Curriculum content and evaluation

Factors		Number of Studies	Percentage of All Studies (n=29)
Evaluations	Staff evaluation only	4	13.8%
	Staff and student evaluation	9	31.0%
	Student evaluation only	16	55.2%
Content Delivery	Lecture	17	58.6%
	Project	20	69.0%
	IHIOS	11	37.9%
	Simulation/case	3	10.3%
	Shadowing	1	3.4%
	Small groups	11	37.9%
QI Curriculum Content	Literature search/benchmarking	4	13.8%
	Failure mode and effects analysis	1	3.4%
	Human factors	2	6.9%
	Systems error/ engineering/practice	3	10.3%
	Patient satisfaction	1	3.4%
	Gap analysis	1	3.4%
	Basic QI	9	31.0%
	PDSA	15	51.7%
	Fishbone diagram	3	10.3%
	Process flow diagrams	6	20.7%
	Audit	5	17.2%
	Lean	2	6.9%
	5 whys	1	3.4%
	Root cause	10	34.5%
	Key stakeholder assessment	4	13.8%
	A3 problem solving	1	3.4%
Curriculum Structure	Mandatory course	15	51.7%
	Elective	6	20.7%
	Standalone program	8	27.6%

4. Discussion

4.1. Themes

In this chapter, we reviewed 29 studies that specifically targeted quality improvement education among medical students from 2009 to 2018. Dates were chosen based on the relevant review by Wong et al. which had searched literature up to January 2009 for both medical students and residents [12]. Other reviews focused solely on patient safety or QI in the clinical setting in both medical students and residents, respectively [13, 14]. The purpose of our systematic review was to provide an update in the literature through December 2018 with a specific focus on medical students' training in quality improvement.

We looked at several factors that included but were not limited to study location (local or international), single or multiple institutions, time of implementation, and delivery. From the results, we were able to derive several themes: driving force for QI training in the USA, current climate in the timing of implementation, multifaceted delivery and use of IHIOS, interprofessional training, organizational change and patient benefits as outcomes, curriculum structure, and number of participants.

The studies included were far reaching but the majority were in the US. This may be a consequence of a particular focus in the US on involving quality improvement in the medical school curriculum. This could be explained by the AAMC developing the Core Entrustable Professional Activities for Entering Residency guideline that contain using quality improvement as a critical competency [3]. The ACGME now includes patient safety and quality improvement in their common requirements for all residency programs so medical schools are likewise responding by adding patient safety and quality improvement into the medical school curriculum.

The best time for the implementation of QI training is not known, although a significant percentage of QI programs are completed during the clinical years. There is a multitude of competing interests during medical school which already contains a full and quick paced curriculum. It would seem natural for medical students to be more preoccupied with learning the basic sciences, anatomy, and physiology rather than learning about QI. In their undergraduate education, students develop a sense of what medical school is and what it means to be a doctor. Their focus is on developing knowledge and clinical skills to care for patients. Clinical years seem a natural time to initiate QI curriculum and projects as this allows for the medical students to have time to acclimate to the demands of medical school and gain some clinical knowledge prior to starting work on QI education or a QI project [40]. However, there has been QI curricula with first year medical students which did demonstrate transfer of knowledge to the clinical context by administering Quality Improvement Knowledge Application Tool- Revised (QIKAT-R), a tool for QI knowledge within a clinical context, and evidence that first-year medical students valued QI lectures [17, 33]. O'Brien et al. described a systems-oriented workplace learning experience for first year medical and pharmacy students where early exposure to system improvement initiatives provided students with realistic experiences that the students will carry with them through future years [43]. In a first-year course studied by Miller et al., responses among medical students were mixed and some did not feel QI information was beneficial early on in training but would be more relevant later on in training [33]. In one pilot study, rising second year students working on QI hospital initiatives were found to be beneficial to both the hospital and the trainees [44].

The curricular delivery was varied amongst the studies with many using a multifaceted program delivery approach [32, 34, 38, 39]. These multifaceted approaches proved to be most effective to introduce different types of learning. Independent modules, reflective writing, group sessions, workshops, faculty mentorship, and individual QI projects provided a well-rounded curriculum where learned skills could then be practiced and implemented [17,40]. Another interesting development since the 2010 study by Wong et al. [12] was the use of the IHIOS [45]. About 37.9% of the studies included used this resource. IHIOS gave students another way to train by having easily accessible standardized training modules that are available on demand to facilitate learning.

Several studies in this review described curricula that showed medical students training with allied health students, nurses, physicians, residents and staff [20, 23, 28]. Many studies have been previously published demonstrating the benefits and obstacles of interprofessional education [20]. Teamwork between interprofessional disciplines can be utilized to address local community issues [4]. In one study, students working on a breastfeeding QI initiative showed a positive behavioral change when they were obligated to work with the different departments and together come up with integrated solutions and recommendations [4].

Many studies in this review went beyond knowledge and satisfaction evaluation. It is interesting to note that all the studies done outside of the US incorporated some form of an experiential component. In fact, 69% of the 29 articles involved some experiential project, a number which was an increase from Wong's previous systematic review.

Organizational change was demonstrated in many of our studies and showed an increase in frequency from past reviews. A study in South Africa revolving around medical students involved in breastfeeding QI resulted in the reinstitution of two hospitals' baby and mother-friendly designation [4]. Students were very proud of their direct involvement in updating the hospital's guidelines. Students in a Tasmanian study had a critical role in improving medical charts which led to an easier means of finding non-compliant patients and proactively connecting with them to improve their care [32]. This clinical audit also provided the general practitioners with new teaching opportunities.

Patient benefits were a key difference from past systematic reviews. 27.6% of our studies had some form of patient benefit experienced while Wong et al. had only two studies showing patient benefits and Kirkman et al. had no studies showing this. This shows an increase in QI projects that actually affect patient satisfaction and health. In one, performance gains were found across patient populations specifically in diabetic foot exams, chlamydia screening, diabetic nephropathy, and use of inhaled steroids for moderate-to-severe persistent asthma [37]. In another study, through their work at a clinical site, a student group improved urine sample collection in first-trimester pregnant patients from 55% to more than 80% [36]. In a third study, three new guidelines were implemented in the emergency departments of three different hospitals [8]. In the 6 months since implementation, there were no patient adverse or serious events to report. In addition, 86% of the departmental providers felt comfortable working with medical students in future emergency department QI projects [8].

The number of participants varies across studies. It is very common to find large numbers during the pre-clinical years with some exceptions. In one study, over a 4-year period, only 22 second year medical students took part in an elective health leadership practicum, representing approximately 5% of students each year [36]. In another one, 23 students had completed a first-year QI and PS elective [41]. In both cases, students participated in an elective. For some studies, it is a very positive development to see a large group of students during clinical years being able to participate in an experiential opportunity [22, 26, 40].

4.2. Challenges and Future Recommendations

Each of these 29 studies noted some challenges and limitations. Bac et al. noted that multiple rotations on the same topic were too long for some of the hospitals and generated fluctuating enthusiasm amongst the student groups [4]. Students also did not have any authority to implement their recommended changes during the QI activity and this was a major constraint in effecting substantial change in some of the institutions [4].

The absence of a clear structure was observed in another study [32]. This study relative to others had a much more difficult time implementing the QI project earlier in the study. Based on Bac et al. and Cox et al. it seems the more structure/direction/responsibilities the medical students were given, the easier the implementation of the QI training was [4, 20].

Frequently, studies were single-site and the sample size was limited, reducing the power of these studies. There were also a few occasions where the medical students in the study were part of an honors program or the QI project was offered as an extracurricular activity [40, 17]. When curriculum is limited to an honors student population or offered on a voluntary basis, there will be inherent selection bias resulting in an underrepresentation of the general medical student population.

A pilot study where 46 students worked on a PDSA project in general practice offices was deemed a success as defined by the students and also by the physicians who made headway in their projects [46]. However, it was a challenge to get the projects done over 4 months with 4–6 dedicated days for their work. Getting started and data access were problems. Curriculum time, resources, and interest are important to the successful completion of QI projects [46]. To maintain enthusiasm, it is also an important element that projects are of interest to both students and the practice.

Variability in curriculum implementation exists. For instance, some studies made the QI curriculum mandatory, whereas others allowed voluntary engagement. All studies gave participants no financial benefit from participation except for one study where students volunteered and were paid a stipend [39]. As different designs were used, not all of the projects performed statistical analysis.

Another limitation is that although students contributed to organizational change, it is not possible to quantitatively measure the student's involvement in organizational change and patient outcome improvements [4]. This was due to the projects being embedded in the context of a complex healthcare setting. There were varying degrees of ownership on the part of the students as their QI project was determined for them [4]. In addition, some hospitals showed little to no interest in the QI projects.

A challenge for systems-oriented workplace learning experiences was identified by O'Brien et al. in the form of support and guidance for the students throughout their healthcare-based experiences [43]. They found that students required exposure to educators within the healthcare system who understood the goals of the medical school. These site leaders were better able to support a successful learning experience for students by identifying the background and structure required, environment conducive to systems-based practice learning, and appropriate scope of work [43]. Headrick et al. found a similar challenge among healthcare sites where many faculty members were unfamiliar with quality improvement initiatives [47].

Sustaining a curriculum was also challenged with finding effective project mentors with adequate quality and safety training [41].

Future directions for QI research should begin to investigate the most beneficial time for initiating QI education [27]. Additionally, identification of the most effective learning technique to implement QI curriculum has not been described. Currently there is evidence of an increased use of multifaceted teaching approaches, but no one or series of techniques have been described as essential or superior. To improve upon past quality improvement studies, future investigations should utilize more quantitative analyses to increase internal and external validity. These future directions will aid in sustaining and further improving upon patient benefits and organizational change for the trainees and the learning environment.

CONCLUSION

This systematic review identified 29 studies that met inclusion criteria. This chapter showed continuous growth beyond medical students' QI knowledge and satisfaction. Organizational change and patient benefit were observed in a majority of the studies. Implementation was across all years of medical education and a variety of educational delivery was implemented. While most studies were from the US, the findings from the different studies are globally relevant.

Major improvements since Wong's systematic review in 2010 were observed. Experiential learning and a longitudinal approach to QI are becoming more common, and the use of IHIOS resources are utilized by several different curricula. Interprofessional training is also increasingly part of QI training. Our investigation indicates that a multimodal curriculum with strong faculty support that occurs longitudinally throughout medical school and that demonstrates direct clinical relevance to the students could provide an effective model for future advancement in QI education.

APPENDIX 1: PUBMED SEARCH STRATEGY

1	"Education, medical"[MeSH Terms] OR "Medical education"[All Fields] OR "Medical students"[All Fields] OR "Medical school"[All Fields]
2	"Quality improvement"[All Fields] OR "Total Quality Management"[All Fields] OR "quality assurance"[All Fields] OR "Health care quality"[All Fields] OR "six sigma"[All Fields] OR "lean principles"[All Fields] OR "root cause analysis"[All Fields] OR PDSA[All Fields]
3	"curriculum"[All Fields] OR "training programs"[All Fields] OR "Learning environment"[All Fields] OR "experiential learning"[All Fields] OR "Clinical performance measures"[All Fields] OR "teaching"[MeSH]
4	1 AND 2 AND 3*
5	AND ("2009/01/01"[PDAT] : "2018/12/31"[PDAT])
6	AND English[lang]
7	NOT (Letter[ptyp] OR Review[ptyp] OR Editorial[ptyp] OR Comment[sb])

*Using parentheses in Basic Search not the Search Builder in Advanced Search.

REFERENCES

[1] Institute of Medicine Committee on Quality of Health Care in America. *Crossing the Quality Chasm: A New Health System for the 21st Century*. Washington (DC): National Academies Press (US).

[2] Institute of Medicine Committee on Quality of Health Care in America. In: Kohn LT, Corrigan JM, Donaldson MS, editors. *To Err is Human: Building a Safer Health System*. Washington (DC): National Academies Press (US); 2000.

[3] Association of American Medical Colleges. *The Core Entrustable Professional Activities (EPAs) for Entering Residency*. https://www.aamc.org/initiatives/coreepas/. Accessed April 30, 2019.

[4] Bac M, Bergh AM, Etsane ME, Hugo J. Medical education and the quality improvement spiral: A case study from Mpumalanga, South Africa. *Afr J Prim Health Care Fam Med*. 2015;7(1).

[5] AAMC. Medical School Graduation Questionnaire. http://www.aamc.org/data/gq/ Cited by: Levitt DS, Hauer KE, Poncelet A, Mookherjee S. An innovative quality improvement

curriculum for third-year medical students. *Med Educ Online.* 2012;17.

[6] Shen B, Dumenco L, Dollase R, George P. The importance of quality improvement education for medical students. *Med Educ.* 2016;50(5):567-8.

[7] Bowser D, Abbas Y, Odunleye T, Broughton E, Bossert T. Pilot study of quality of care training and knowledge in Sub-Saharan African medical schools. *Int J Med Educ.* 2017;8:276-82.

[8] Manning MW, Bean EW, Miller AC, Templer SJ, Mackenzie RS, Richardson DM, et al. Using medical student quality improvement projects to promote evidence-based care in the emergency department. *West J Emerg Med.* 2018;19(1):148-57.

[9] *Accreditation Council for Graduate Medical Education (ACGME). Common Program Requirements.* https://acgme.org/What-We-Do/Accreditation/Common-Program-Requirements. Accessed April 30, 2019.

[10] *Accreditation Council for Graduate Medical Education (ACGME). Clinical Learning Environment Review (CLER).* https://www.acgme.org/What-We-Do/Initiatives/Clinical-Learning-Environment-Review-CLER. Accessed April 30, 2019.

[11] Bergh AM, Bac M, Hugo J, Sandars J. "Making a difference"-Medical students' opportunities for transformational change in health care and learning through quality improvement projects. *BMC Med Educ.* 2016;16:171.

[12] Wong BM, Etchells EE, Kuper A, Levinson W, Shojania KG. Teaching quality improvement and patient safety to trainees: A systematic review. *Acad Med.* 2010;85(9):1425-39.

[13] Kirkman MA, Sevdalis N, Arora S, Baker P, Vincent C, Ahmed M. The outcomes of recent patient safety education interventions for trainee physicians and medical students: a systematic review. *BMJ Open.* 2015;5(5):e007705.

[14] Jones AC, Shipman SA, Ogrinc G. Key characteristics of successful quality improvement curricula in physician education: a realist review. *BMJ Qual Saf.* 2015;24(1):77-88.

[15] Bartlett CS, Huerta SA. Creating change: an experiential quality improvement and patient safety curriculum for medical students. *MedEdPORTAL*. 2018;14:10660.

[16] Bradham TS, Sponsler KC, Watkins SC, Ehrenfeld JM. Creating a quality improvement course for undergraduate medical education: practice what you teach. *Acad Med*. 2018;93(10):1491-6.

[17] Brown A, Nidumolu A, Stanhope A, Koh J, Greenway M, Grierson L. Can first-year medical students acquire quality improvement knowledge prior to substantial clinical exposure? A mixed-methods evaluation of a pre-clerkship curriculum that uses education as the context for learning. *BMJ Qual Saf*. 2018;27(7):576-82.

[18] Burnett E, Davey P, Gray N, Tully V, Breckenridge J. Medical students as agents of change: a qualitative exploratory study. *BMJ Open Qual*. 2018;7(3):e000420.

[19] Chen CA, Park RJ, Hegde JV, Jun T, Christman MP, Yoo SM, et al. How we used a patient visit tracker tool to advance experiential learning in systems-based practice and quality improvement in a medical student clinic. *Med Teach*. 2016;38(1):36-40.

[20] Cox KR, Scott SD, Hall LW, Aud MA, Headrick LA, Madsen R. Uncovering differences among health professions trainees exposed to an interprofessional patient safety curriculum. *Qual Manag Health Care*. 2009;18(3):182-93.

[21] Dumenco L, Monteiro K, George P, McNicoll L, Warrier S, Dollase R. An interactive quality improvement and patient safety workshop for first-year medical students. *MedEdPORTAL*. 2018;14:10734.

[22] Dysinger WS, Pappas JM. A fourth-year medical school rotation in quality, patient safety, and population medicine. *Am J Prev Med*. 2011;41(4 Suppl 3):S200-5.

[23] Elghouche AN, Lobo BC, Wannemuehler TJ, Johnson KE, Matt BH, Woodward-Hagg HK, et al. Lean Belt certification: pathway for student, resident, and faculty development and scholarship. *Otolaryngol Head Neck Surg*. 2016;154(5):785-8.

[24] Hall LW, Headrick LA, Cox KR, Deane K, Gay JW, Brandt J. Linking health professional learners and health care workers on action-based improvement teams. *Qual Manag Health Care*. 2009;18(3):194-201.

[25] Huntington JT, Dycus P, Hix C, West R, McKeon L, Coleman MT, et al. A standardized curriculum to introduce novice health professional students to practice-based learning and improvement: a multi-institutional pilot study. *Qual Manag Health Care*. 2009;18(3):174-81.

[26] Jackson B, Chandauka R, Vivekananda-Schmidt P. Introducing quality improvement teaching into general practice undergraduate placements. *Educ Prim Care*. 2018;29(4):228-31.

[27] James TA, Goedde M, Bertsch T, Beatty D. Advancing the future of patient safety in oncology: implications of patient safety education on cancer care delivery. *J Cancer Educ*. 2016;31(3):488-92.

[28] Kool B, Wise MR, Peiris-John R, Sadler L, Mahony F, Wells S. Is the delivery of a quality improvement education programme in obstetrics and gynaecology for final year medical students feasible and still effective in a shortened time frame? *BMC Med Educ*. 2017;17(1).

[29] Kutaimy R, Zhang L, Blok D, Kelly R, Kovacevic N, Levoska M, et al. Integrating patient safety education into early medical education utilizing cadaver, sponges, and an inter-professional team. *BMC Med Educ*. 2018;18(1):215.

[30] Levitt DS, Hauer KE, Poncelet A, Mookherjee S. An innovative quality improvement curriculum for third-year medical students. *Med Educ Online*. 2012;17.

[31] Margalit R, Thompson S, Visovsky C, Geske J, Collier D, Birk T, et al. From professional silos to interprofessional education: campuswide focus on quality of care. *Qual Manag Health Care*. 2009;18(3):165-73.

[32] Mauldon E, Radford J, Todd A. Expanding capacity for supervision in general practice through student-engaged clinical audit. *Qual Prim Care*. 2014;22(1):35-41.

[33] Miller R, Winterton T, Hoffman WW. Building a whole new mind: an interprofessional experience in patient safety and quality improvement

education using the IHI Open School. *S D Med.* 2014;67(1):17-9, 21-3.

[34] Miller RJ, Hoffman WW. "Heart Bone"--the case for the IHI Open School as connector: a model for integrating quality improvement and patient safety into health professions curricula. *S D Med.* 2015;68(6):245-50.

[35] Mookherjee S, Ranji S, Neeman N, Sehgal N. An advanced quality improvement and patient safety elective. *Clin Teach.* 2013;10(6):368-73.

[36] Ogrinc G, Nierenberg DW, Batalden PB. Building experiential learning about quality improvement into a medical school curriculum: the Dartmouth experience. *Health Aff (Millwood).* 2011;30(4):716-22.

[37] O'Neill SM, Henschen BL, Unger ED, Jansson PS, Unti K, Bortoletto P, et al. Educating future physicians to track health care quality: feasibility and perceived impact of a health care quality report card for medical students. *Acad Med.* 2013;88(10):1564-9.

[38] Paxton JH, Rubinfeld IS. Medical errors education: a prospective study of a new educational tool. *Am J Med Qual.* 2010;25(2):135-42.

[39] Sweigart JR, Tad YD, Pierce R, Wagner E, Glasheen JJ. The Health Innovations Scholars Program: a model for accelerating preclinical medical students' mastery of skills for leading improvement of clinical systems. *Am J Med Qual.* 2016;31(4):293-300.

[40] Tartaglia KM, Walker C. Effectiveness of a quality improvement curriculum for medical students. *Med Educ Online.* 2015;20:27133.

[41] Vinci LM, Oyler J, Arora VM. The quality and safety track: training future physician leaders. *Am J Med Qual.* 2014;29(4):277-83.

[42] Praslova L. Adaptation of Kirkpatrick's four level model of training criteria to assessment of learning outcomes and program evaluation in higher education. *Educational Assessment, Evaluation and Accountability.* 2010;22(3):215-225.

[43] O'Brien BC, Bachhuber MR, Teherani A, Iker TM, Batt J, O'Sullivan PS. Systems-oriented workplace learning experiences for early learners: three models. *Acad Med.* 2017;92(5):684-93.

[44] Brannan GD, Russ R, Winemiller TR, Mast E. Linking community hospital initiatives with osteopathic medical students' quality improvement training: a pilot program. *J Am Osteopath Assoc*, 2016;116(1):36-41.

[45] Institute for Healthcare Improvement. Open School. http://www.ihi.org/education/IHIOpenSchool/Pages/default.aspx. Accessed April 30, 2019.

[46] Wylie A, Leedham-Green K. Piloting quality improvement projects in undergraduate medical education. *Med Educ*. 2017;51(5):543-544.

[47] Headrick LA, Barton AJ, Ogrinc G, et al. Results of an effort to integrate quality and safety into medical and nursing school curricula and foster joint learning. *Health Aff (Millwood)*. 2012;31(12):2669-2680.

Reviewed by: Godwin Dogbey, PhD, Biostatistician, Campbell University School of Osteopathic Medicine, Buies Creek, NC, US.

In: Exploring the Opportunities ...
Editor: Elias A. Jespersen

ISBN: 978-1-53616-213-4
© 2019 Nova Science Publishers, Inc.

Chapter 2

EXPERIENTIAL RESEARCH AND SCHOLARLY PROGRAMS FOR MEDICAL STUDENTS: SHORT-TERM PARADIGMS

Clarissa Dass[1], DO, Melissa Ianitelli[1], DO, David Tolentino[2], DO, Jody Gerome[3], DO, Nicole Wadsworth[4], DO and Grace D. Brannan[5],*, PhD

[1]Department of Cardiovascular Disease,
McLaren Macomb Hospital, Mount Clemens, MI, US
[2]Department of Clinical Affairs, Campbell University
School of Medicine, Buies Creek, NC, US
[3]Department of Academic Affairs, Ohio University
Heritage College of Osteopathic Medicine, OH, US
[4]Department of Academic Affairs, New York College of
Osteopathic Medicine, New York, US
[5]GDB Research and Statistical Consulting, Athens, OH, US

---

* Corresponding Author's Email: gracebrannan2013@gmail.com.

Abstract

The decline in physician scientists has prompted attention from the medical field. With increasing focus on evidence-based medicine, there is an ongoing need to enhance research education for medical trainees. The undergraduate medical profession has recognized the need with the development of Entrustable Professional Activity or EPA by the Association of American Medical Colleges. Specifically, EPA 7 speaks to evidence-based medicine which is rooted in research and scholarly skills. This puts additional emphasis on research during medical school. To further highlight the importance of research, The Accreditation Council for Graduate Medical Education, the accrediting body for residency, requires that residents participate in research and scholarly activities. As such, it is very critical that medical students are equipped with research skills and experience to effectively meet residency requirements. Where schools may be challenged is providing experiential or hands-on opportunities. Some schools have added a fifth year to include research projects as a critical component. Dual degrees such as an MD/PhD and DO/PhD are also common. However, not all medical students will have the opportunity or interest to engage in these long-term programs. The objective of this chapter was to describe the curricula and analyze results from two short term programs: a Summer Research and Scholarly Program between the first and second year of medical school and Research Rotation Electives offered to third- and fourth- year students.

This chapter describes an IRB-approved study which involved a retrospective review of data accumulated over several years. Descriptive data was generated and analyzed. Student participation in both programs increased over the years. Students were statistically significantly ($p=0.00001$) mentored by more physicians compared to research scientists. There were subsequently significantly more students in both programs involved in clinical studies ($p=0.00001$). Participation by gender was not significantly different for summer ($p=0.372$) or elective participants ($p=0.105$). Summer researchers were mostly involved in data collection while elective students were increasingly involved in other activities such as proposal development and also took on more responsibility ($p=0.00001$). The increase noted in both programs and the equal participation of female and male medical students were very encouraging. We also described the curricula to provide detail to readers who are creating their own curriculum on short-term programs to provide hands-on research opportunities for students.

Keywords: research and scholarly experience, medical students, summer research, research rotation elective, EPA, ACGME

1. INTRODUCTION

In 1910, the Flexner Report or "Medical Education in the United States and Canada" was written by Abraham Flexner, a research scholar at the Carnegie Foundation [1]. The Flexner Report assessed the medical education system through all of the 155 medical schools at that time. The Flexner report advocated for formal analytic training while also stressing the importance of conducting research during medical school to help strengthen patient care. However, it was not until the mid-1950s that research during medical school fully developed [2]. However, many studies have shown that there is a decline in the number of "physician-scientists" in the United States each year, which could be partially attributed to inconsistent training in medical school towards research.

Involvement in research in medical school allows for a strong educational and career foundation for medical students. It allows for development of students' skills as physicians by strengthening critical thinking and forming analytical skills to stay updated on medical literature while also performing evidence-based medicine [3]. Performing research during medical school also helps foster medical students' interest in academic medical careers and postgraduate research [4]. Studies found that medical students who conducted research during medical school were more than three times as likely to perform research in their careers as physicians [5].

The medical profession has recognized the need and stepped up to the plate with several developments. The Association of American Medical Colleges' (AAMC) Entrustable Professional Activity (EPA) outlines minimum characteristics for a student to qualify for residency [6]. EPA 7 speaks to evidence-based medicine which is rooted in research and scholarly skills, but are usually delivered in didactic lectures. The AAMC collected information on first year residents by specialty and found that the number of research experiences range from 1.5-4.5 while the number of abstracts, presentations, and publications range from 2.2-15.8, depending on the specialty [7]. These outcomes were accumulated not only during the first year of residency but during and prior to medical school. This puts additional emphasis on research during medical school.

To further highlight the importance of research, The Accreditation Council for Graduate Medical Education (ACGME), which accredits medical residencies in the United States, requires that residents participate in research and scholarly activities [8]. In fact, on an annual basis, ACGME collects information on residents' ongoing projects and completed outcomes such as publications and poster and oral presentations. This emphasis demonstrates that it is critical that medical students are equipped with research skills and experience to effectively meet residency requirements.

A literature review completed in 2013 found that the most common fields of medicine in which research was performed by medical students included but were not limited to, Psychiatry, General Medicine, and Community Medicine [4]. Medical students were more likely to perform research in their desired fields of training and the most common reason for conducting research in medical school was found to be career progression and increasing competitiveness of their residency application [5]. Other factors that were found to influence research during medical school included previous research experience, academic success, having an advanced degree at the time of enrollment, and financial components [5].

At this time, a consistent curriculum at medical schools throughout the United States for research does not exist [5]. There are a variety of routes that students can take to conduct research including summer research electives, mandatory study modules, independent research activities or dual-degree programs. Research opportunities and expectations are strongly dependent on the requirements of the medical schools. For example, one medical school allows students to participate in research during their third year of training while in another, medical students conduct research projects throughout the four years of medical school [9].

According to a survey by the Liaison Committee on Medical Education conducted between 2016 and 2017, 62 of 145 medical schools were found to have a research requirement for MD students [10]. About 68% of schools formally supported students to take a non-degree research year [3]. A variety of reasons have been formulated for taking a non-degree research year including to gain research training without pursuing dual degree program, such as MD/PhD or DO/PhD, to pursue academic interest or as a graduation requirement. However, the most common reason that has been found for pursuing a non-degree research year is to increase the competitiveness of the student's application for residency [3].

In the United States, the National Institute of Health Medical Scientist Training Program provides grants and funding to medical schools for dual-training programs, such as MD/PhD [11]. These programs provide medical students with dedicated years outside of their medical training to conduct biomedical research. There are currently 50 programs with approximately 970 trainees. The average length of these programs is about 8 years. Studies have shown that these programs have been successful in training physician-scientists with 81% of MD/PhD graduates in academic positions and 82% of graduates performing research. However, only 3% of the medical student population are from these dual-training programs [4].

Where many schools are challenged is providing experiential or hands-on opportunities within a shorter timeframe to make research accessible and interesting to the greater majority of medical students. Afterall, all students must be trained in research to prepare them for the rigors of scholarly requirements in residency. The objective of this chapter was to describe the curricula and analyze results from two short term programs from a single institution: a summer research and scholarly program and research rotation electives.

2. PROGRAM DESCRIPTION

2.1. Summer Research and Scholarly Program

2.1.1. Description

The summer between year 1 and year 2 provides an ideal time for students to explore research. There are several programs available to students that are internal and external to Ohio University (OU). At OU Heritage College of Osteopathic Medicine (HCOM), a summer program geared towards basic science experience has been in existence for decades. The impetus for this complementary, voluntary summer program is to focus on clinical research opportunities [12]. In addition, the program provides a structure to ensure that students participating in internal and external scholarly opportunities obtain proper ethics approval prior to starting their research.

2.1.2. Structure and Evolution

The students registered their participation with the Research Education Office and gained approval from the Associate Dean of Academic Affairs. Approvals would occur once the student had completed all appropriate training, met institutional requirements, completed human subjects or animal training, obtained Institutional Review Board (IRB) or Institutional Animal Care and Use Committee (IACUC) approval or demonstrated reciprocity and completed an orientation. Although intensive from an administrative standpoint, this process ensured that research was approved, and appropriate documents were in place before the project started.

2.1.3. Program Goal

To provide medical students starting in 2013 with early research and scholarly experiential opportunities, basic ethics training and a mechanism to ensure that appropriate documents were in place prior to starting the project.

2.1.4. Program Components

Students participated in many different types of research activities. The types of programs available to students included: programs created with partner hospitals, national programs we or the student found as part of our search for available programs, and research opportunities with faculty at HCOM. These opportunities were sometimes funded and sometimes voluntary in nature. Programs were in a variety of locations, both locally and nationally. Time commitment ranged from 8-10 weeks.

Several months prior, we advertised all opportunities to students and provided information that describes the approval process and documents they must complete if they have found an opportunity on their own. To facilitate the process, we worked with the university's Office of Research Compliance to create a deferral process for projects occurring outside the institution.

The programs in which the students participated varied greatly and included bench research, clinical research, acquiring data for ongoing projects as well as opportunities for exposure to patient care as part of the research or as a separate component.

2.1.5. Personnel

The Research Education Office, the Predoctoral Office, Academic Affairs, and the university Office of Research Compliance were involved in the process.

2.1.6. Registration and Selection of Medical Students

Students self-selected to participate in this program. In some cases, opportunities were competitive, and students had to have been selected by the mentor or project sponsor. Participants must have been in good standing with HCOM and have successfully completed the first year of medical school.

2.1.7. Expectations and Outcomes

As this was a voluntary, not for credit program, our focus was on providing opportunities and ensuring ethical documents are in place before the opportunity commenced. The expectations and outcomes were: students met institutional (OU and host institution) requirements; completed human subjects/animal training, if applicable; and, completed the experience. They also attended orientation about professional and ethical conduct.

2.2. Research Rotation Electives

2.2.1. Description

The Research Rotation Electives were launched in 2005 as a scholarly opportunity for third- and fourth- year students [12]. It is a graded elective. The electives were expanded in 2008 into 4 categories to better serve the specific needs of students: (1) introduction to research, 1 week; (2) case report, up to 3 weeks; (3) literature review, up to 3 weeks; and (4) retrospective, prospective, and meta-analysis research, 3 to 12 weeks.

2.2.2. Program Goal

The overall goal of the elective is to provide an experiential research and scholarly opportunity with protected time within a structured curriculum. Rotation objectives pertaining to the knowledge and skills domain are specified for each rotation (e.g., state a research hypothesis, conduct a critical literature review, write a proposal, collect data in an ethical manner, interpret results, etc.).

2.2.3. Individual Rotation Description

Each elective is structured differently to provide the best experience for the student. Topics are chosen by the student, mentor or both. Other than the Introduction to Research, which takes place on main campus, the other research electives can take place anywhere, even outside of the country, as long as the proper documents are in place.

2.2.3.1. Introduction to Research

This rotation is geared towards any student who do not have prior research or scholarly experience. The instructors provided a broad overview of research via didactics, observations, and hands-on activities on a variety of topics including critical review of the literature, research methods, life cycle of a research study, human and animal subject protection, shadowing a researcher, development of a research protocol, introduction to statistics, funding and resources, budget creation, and dissemination. This course takes place on the main campus. As the final paper is a literature review, it does not require prior IRB approval.

Rotation Objectives:

- State a research hypothesis
- Define research/project objectives
- Effectively review the literature
- Determine the components of a research protocol
- Explain the importance of required documents, determine when needed, and describe the processes involved
- Understand and identify funding sources and the importance of budget creation
- Describe the process involved in proper, ethical, and legal collection of data or information
- Understand the importance of translating the results of the study into a more practical or actionable outcome and the implications of the study outcome
- Understand and be able to justify the importance of a study and its contribution to evidence-based medicine
- Understand the process of disseminating research findings

2.2.3.2. Critical Literature Review

This rotation provides an introduction to critical review of literature via hands-on experience. An IRB approval is not required. Identifying a mentor and an appropriate topic are a pre-requisite to enrollment in this course. Deliverables are due within 2 weeks of the end of the rotation.

Rotation Objectives:

- Define/state research objective(s)
- Effectively review the literature
- List variables/factors to be studied that will provide an answer to objectives
- Explain the importance of required documents

- Determine inclusion/exclusion criteria to be applied to selecting relevant studies
- Translate the results of the study into a more practical or actionable outcome

2.2.3.3. Case-Based Study

This rotation provides an opportunity to write a case report, which is defined as a description of the symptoms, diagnosis, treatment, and follow-up of a patient related to a rare or unusual course of events. A case report consists of one case or multiple cases ($N \leq 3$).

Finding an acceptable case to report is a pre-requisite for enrollment in the Case-Based Study research rotation; the rotation is not intended to be used to locate a case on which to report. An initial review of the literature is required to provide the necessary justification the case report would offer new/valuable information to the body of knowledge in the subject area. If the subject area is already rich with information on similar cases, then the proposed case would be rejected as a case report for this rotation.

Rotation Objectives:

- Effectively review the literature
- Determine the objective of the case study
- Identify a target journal for publication and follow submission guidelines
- Explain the importance of required documents, determine when needed, and describe the processes involved
- Describe the process involved in the proper and legal collection of data or information
- Translate the results of the case study into a more practical or actionable outcome
- Discuss the implications of the study outcome
- Complete and present a poster and/or submit a manuscript for publication in a peer-reviewed journal

- Justify the importance of the study and its contribution to evidence-based medicine
- Effectively work with the preceptor and the Research Education Office in accomplishing all goals

2.2.3.4. Retrospective, Prospective and Meta-Analysis Studies

Student research for this rotation consists of any of the following types of studies: a chart review, an animal study, bench research, a survey study, or a meta-analysis, to name a few. To accomplish this, this rotation provides a hands-on experience.

To achieve the rotation objectives, the student is expected to significantly contribute to several if not all of the following research concepts or steps: identify gaps in the current treatment, diagnosis and management of patients, develop research question and objectives, choose appropriate research design, statistics and hypothesis testing, human subject protection, proposal development, and dissemination of scientific findings as a means of contributing to evidence-based medicine.

The initial weeks of the Retrospective, Prospective, and Meta-Analysis Studies research rotation (up to six) could be used for lecture and discussion-type instructions and development of the research proposal. For human subjects' research an IRB review and approval of the proposal was required. Prior to submitting any materials to a hospital compliance officer or research office, students are required to contact the college's Research Education Office.

Students may apply for a second block of time which would be contingent upon several factors such as successfully clearing the university's Office of Research Compliance and meeting all goals for the first block. Typically, this second block of time is used to initiate the study's protocol, gather data, perform data analyses, and/or prepare a final manuscript.

Rotation Objectives:

- Define/state a research hypothesis and objectives
- Effectively review the literature
- Write a research protocol

- List variables/factors to be studied that will provide an answer to objectives and explain the process of choosing a research design
- Explain the importance of required documents
- Determine inclusion/exclusion criteria to be applied to selecting study participants and/or studies to be included in the review
- Describe the process involved in proper and legal collection of data or information
- Translate the results of the study into a more practical or actionable outcome
- Comprehend statistical results, discuss the implications of the study outcome, justify the importance of the study and its contribution to evidence-based medicine
- Complete and present a poster and/or submit a manuscript for publication in a peer-reviewed journal

There were some limitations in the organization of this rotation. While the length of this rotation was very flexible (3-12 weeks), twelve weeks is the maximum allotted for the Retrospective, Prospective, and Meta-Analysis Studies research rotation. The twelve weeks do not need to be completed consecutively. In fact, the time could be divided across two adjacent academic years (e.g., six weeks in the third-year and six weeks in the fourth-year). This flexibility allows more convenience of scheduling for the medical student. However, if the initial weeks of this research elective are used for didactic instruction and development of the research proposal (a maximum of six weeks), then only six weeks of protected time remain for the student to complete all the required activities and deliverables, compelling the student to continue the research truly as a part of a longitudinal experience concurrently with other rotations. Second, recognizing Retrospective, Prospective, and Meta-Analysis Studies could be time- and labor-intensive, a student's last opportunity to enroll in this particular research elective rotation is one semester prior to graduation. This stipulation in procedure is to ensure the completion of assignments and deliverables did not jeopardize a student's graduation status.

2.2.4. Process

The application process for this rotation provides an opportunity to set and clarify expectations, answer questions and define roles, assess skill level and experience, and anticipate and proactively resolve problems. The student is mandated to meet with the college's Research Education Office prior to registration for this rotation. This meeting serves as an opportunity for the student to discuss past research experiences and personal objectives for the rotation with the goal of ensuring a rewarding and successful rotation. The following are some of the details that need clarification:

- Specific student responsibilities on the rotation
- Specific expectations of the student on the rotation
- Goals, objectives, structure, timeline, and expected measurable outcomes and deliverables of the rotation
- Required rotation assignments (e.g., data collection, protocol development, presentation of results to conferences and research days, submission of manuscript to peer reviewed journal, co-authorship)
- Subsequent follow-up meeting times to provide student performance feedback

Students use an online registration and self-select for the elective. To be able to participate, the student must be in good academic standing, has the elective rotation time to complete the rotation, and does not have any prior professional infractions.

2.2.5. Personnel

This program involves the Mentor, Research Education Office, Predoctoral Clinical Office, and the university Office of Research Compliance (in projects where this is applicable).

2.2.6. Expectations and Deliverables

Students are expected to provide two deliverables: 1) a final scholarly paper and 2) a 3 to 5-page reflection paper based on their experiences during the rotation. In addition, satisfactory completion of the following is required to receive credit for this rotation:

- Meeting all objectives and deliverables identified within the timeframe of the rotation
- Submission of individual preceptor and student evaluations of the rotation
- Submission of all requirements/deliverables (including the reflection/summative paper describing the work performed during the timeframe of the rotation in relation to the learning objectives) to the preceptor, Research Education Office, and predoctoral clinical office.

3. METHODS

This chapter describes a study approved by the Ohio University Institutional Review Board (OU16-E-319). A retrospective review of the data for the Summer Research and Scholarly Program and Research Rotation Electives was conducted. IBM SPSS Statistics for Windows, Version 25.0 (IBM Corp., Armonk, NY) was used to analyze the data. Descriptive statistics were generated. Where appropriate, inferential analyses were performed. Statistical significance was set at a p value < .05.

4. RESULTS

4.1. Summer Research Outcomes

All students reported in this chapter met the requirements prior to engaging in each scholarly experience. All students also completed the programs. A total of 152 student participated between 2013 and 2016. The summer research participation statistically significantly (p=0.001) increased during these years (Table 1). Although there was a slightly higher number of male than female students, there was no statistical significance between the two values (Table 2). The number of physician mentors were significantly higher than scientists (p=0.00001).

Table 1. Number of summer research participants per year

Participation Year	Frequency	Percent	p value*
2013	24	15.8	0.001
2014	28	18.4	
2015	52	34.2	
2016	48	31.6	
Total	152	100	

*p value was across all years.

Table 2. Demographic information of summer research participants and mentors

Category	Frequency	Percent	p value*
Gender			
F	70	46.1	0.37200
M	82	53.9	
Total	152	100	
Mentor			
MD, DO	117	77	0.00001
PhD, MS, MS/RD, PharmD	35	23	
Total	152	100	

*p value was across gender or mentor.

Writing, data collection, proposal development for submission to the IRB, and literature review were the activities students were involved in (Table 3). Students significantly reported being involved in data collection than other activities listed (p=0.00001). Clinical or community health projects were significantly the most common type of research (p=0.00001). A small cohort of students were involved in medical education research.

Table 3. Summer research participants type of research and activity

Category	Frequency*	Percent	p value**
Activity			
Writing	8	5.3	0.00001
Data collection	118	78.7	
Proposal development (IRB)	16	10.7	
Literature review	8	5.3	
Total	150	100	
Type of Research			
Clinical, community health	127	83.6	0.00001
Bench or animal, engineering, biomechanics	21	13.8	
Medical education	4	2.6	
Total	152	100	
Type of Clinical/Human Subject Research			
Case report case series	8	6.2	0.00001
Critical literature review	8	6.2	
Randomized controlled trial	3	2.3	
Cohort, cross sectional, and case control	111	85.4	
Total	130	100	

*reflects missing data.
**p value was calculated across activity, type of research or clinical research.

Majority of the students (85%) were involved in non-experimental type of studies such as cohort, cross-sectional, and case control (p=0.00001). Very few students were involved in randomized controlled studies which is expected for the level of medical and research training they were at this point in their education. This is a function of the short time a student spends on an individual project. Most students want to be involved from project inception to publication, which is difficult to achieve in a randomized controlled study.

4.2. Research Rotation Elective Outcomes

Over an 11-year period, from Academic Year July 2005-June 2006 to July 2015-June 2016, student participation in the elective statistically significantly increased (p=0.001) (Table 4). Part of this increase is based on the interest built during the research participation during the summer when they were rising second year students.

Table 4. Number of research rotation elective participants per academic year

Academic Year	Frequency	Percent	p value*
July 2005-June 2006	7	5.1	0.00001
July 2006-June 2007	5	3.6	
July 2007-June 2008	4	2.9	
July 2008- June 2009	9	6.5	
July 2009- June 2010	9	6.5	
July 2010- June 2011	8	5.8	
July 2011-June 2012	7	5.1	
July 2012- June 2013	19	13.8	
July 2013- June 2014	22	15.9	
July 2014-June 2015	18	13	
July 2015-June 2016	30	21.7	
Total	138	100	

*p value was calculated across years.

Table 5. Demographic information of research rotation participants and mentors

Category	Frequency	Percent	p value*
Training Year			
Third	41	29.7	0.00001
Fourth	97	70.3	
Total	138	100	
Gender			
F	79	57.2	0.105
M	59	42.8	
Total	138	100	
Mentor			
MD, DO	105	76.1	0.0001
PhD, MS, MS/RD, PharmD	33	23.9	
Total	138	100	

*p value was calculated across training year, gender or mentor.

A significantly higher number of fourth year students than third year students ((p=0.00001) participate in research. This is likely due to schedule flexibility in the fourth year student curriculum, which allows for more student choice. Although there was a higher number of male than female students, there was no statistical significance between the two values (Table

5). Similar to summer research students, there were significantly more physician mentors than scientists (p=0.0001).

Table 6. Research rotation elective participants' type of research and activity

Category	Frequency	Percent	p value*
Research Activity			
Writing	14	10.1	0.00001
Data analysis and modeling	7	5.1	
Data collection	59	42.8	
Proposal development (IRB and grant)	26	18.8	
Literature review	13	9.4	
Combination skills	19	13.8	
Total	138	100	
Type of Research			
Clinical, community health	113	81.9	0.00001
Bench or animal, engineering, biomechanics	18	13	
Introduction to Research	2	1.4	
Medical education	5	3.6	
Total	138	100	
Type of Clinical/Human Subject Research			
Case report or case series	11	9.4	0.00001
Critical literature review	17	14.5	
Randomized controlled trial	17	14.5	
Cohort, cross sectional and case control	71	60.7	
Meta-analysis	1	0.9	
Total	117	100	

*p value was calculated across activity, type of research or clinical research.

Writing, data collection, proposal development for submission to the IRB, and literature review were the same activities students were involved in (Table 6). However, the proportion has changed. Similar to the summer research students, research rotation elective students are significantly involved in data collection than other activities, but proposal development and writing also increased in proportion (p=0.00001). In addition, data analysis and combination activities, meaning being involved in more than one activity, also were added to the list. Similar to summer research, clinical or community health projects were significantly the most common type of research (p=0.00001). In addition, there were two students who participated in the Introduction to Research elective.

Majority of the students (61%) were involved in non-experimental type of studies such as cohort, cross-sectional, and case control (p=0.00001).

5. DISCUSSION

5.1. Increase in Research Interest

From 1980 to 2010, there was a significant increase in medical student research [4]. This also is the same trend observed in our two scholarly programs. This is a positive development considering that the number of physician scientists who claim research as their primary career has declined significantly since the 1980s [13]. Similarly, the number of medical school professors who participated in research as evidenced by being principal investigator on NIH grants also significantly declined from the 1980s [13].

Scholarly programs such as described in this chapter are a means to expose students to scholarly activities. Students who participated in research during medical school were found to have a higher likelihood of being involved in short term and even academic careers later [5]. However, even programs which provide in-depth experiential opportunities in addition to a standard research curriculum have challenges related to the lack of a standardized structure and therefore are hard to evaluate in terms of effectiveness [14]. In addition, long term impact is even more difficult to assess [14].

Evidence-based medicine is rooted in research and early exposure such as during the Summer Program could instill these skills and mindset early on. Studies have shown that teaching the importance and basics of evidence-based medicine and research during medical school positively influences post-graduate interest in research and understanding of research-based medicine [15]. For instance, the ability to publish research as a medical student has been shown to strongly influence a medical student's chance at achieving a more competitive residency while also providing stronger academic achievements in the classroom and in the research field [15]. The field and practice of medicine is also strongly influenced by evidence based medicine with its ability to combine individual clinical expertise with the best available scientific evidence from the literature.

Implementing scholarly programs rely on several critical factors such as administrative support, solid mentorship, and structure that supports the specific needs of students [14]. Training in clinical research, research infrastructure, not having enough time, inadequate scientific writing skills, and lack of access to assistance were some of the needs expressed in prior studies [16]. The two programs described in this chapter are two of many possible models to alleviate these barriers.

5.2. Gender

In this chapter, we found no statistical difference in medical student research involvement based on gender for both programs. A study in 2015 found the same results [5]. These are very encouraging since an earlier study that analyzed data collected from the Association of American Medical Colleges, Howard Hughes Medical Institute and National Institute of Health evaluated further the gender gap in research between 1978 and 1996, which revealed there was a consistently smaller percentage of women than men who expressed strong research intentions with a statistical significant difference in 1988, 1989 and 1991, and female graduating medical students also showed less interest in research driven careers [17].

5.3. Research Category

It is not surprising that there were only 13.8% of students involved in bench or basic science research during summer. This summer program is complementary to another scholarly fellowship program at the medical college which focused on opportunities in this type of research. The fellowship program is an opportunity for students to participate in either basic science or clinical research but since it is on main campus, there were usually more basic science research opportunities available.

Similar to an earlier study on trends of published research by students, clinical and community health research were the predominant types with medical education research occurring less than these two [4]. In terms of human subjects' research, according to a literature review, the most common types of studies completed by medical students were review articles, cross-sectional studies, case reports, case control studies, and cohort studies [4].

5.4. Type of Research Activity

The increase in variety of research activities during third- and fourth-year research rotation elective could point to the fact that students increased their skills and comfort level from when they were engaged in summer research as rising second year students. There also was a notable increase in involvement in randomized controlled studies and a meta-analysis. Perhaps this is a reflection of the student's better understanding of the complexity of research design and development.

Globally, medical students were found to be interested in research but do not have the necessary skills [16]. Programs such as summer research leading into a research rotation opportunity afford the students the ability to gain these skills longitudinally.

In one study, a survey completed by medical students revealed that after completion of their research projects, the majority were able to develop new research questions, analyze data, develop study methodology, review literature and write a manuscript. According to surveyed faculty, medical students were found to be of most assistance in collecting data and data analysis [18].

5.5. Mentor

For both programs, it was common for students to choose mentors who are clinical physicians due to interest in their individual fields or the opportunity to work with patients. Additionally, many students aim for publication in their field of interest, and clinical faculty can support this endeavor.

In an article describing several scholarly concentration programs, challenges such as lack of rigor in projects conducted were discussed [19]. One factor that however contributes to the programs' success was research mentorship, which is critical in providing role models for students on how to integrate practice, research and teaching which may help increase the number of trainees interested in academic pathways.

Only a small fraction of students were involved in medical education research in both programs. This is definitely an area that needs improvement. It has been demonstrated that trainees who were exposed to medical educator mentors and engage in educational scholarly work are more predisposed to pursue an academic career than those who were not [20]. Introducing students to medical education research early on may be one way to help reverse trainees' growing disinterest in academic medicine.

5.6. Year Research Is Conducted

In a given year, more students participated in summer research than in a research rotation elective. This is due to the fact that summer between the first and second year is considered as a free and unstructured period during medical school. During the third and fourth years, other electives are also in competition with the research elective. In one school, a longitudinal program over the first two years of medical school was utilized [21]. The program started with didactics and culminated with a mentored project in one of nine areas of medical scholarship. While the program has been successful, challenges such as protected time in a very packed curriculum and the need for dedicated administrative support were encountered.

5.7. Limitations

The outcomes we measured and reported in this chapter were limited to the number of participants, the type of skills acquired, the type of mentors, the type of research undertaken, and the completion of pre-requisite documents and the program for the summer research. We did not track indicators such as publications and presentations. A systematic review of scholarly concentration programs and medical student research productivity also found similar trends of programs being challenged with tracking outcomes [14]. However, they only tracked programs that provided an in-depth scholarly experience beyond the core curriculum, longer than a summer experience and not dual-degree tracks (e.g., MD/PhD programs).

The limitations of these research programs were determined by availability of opportunities. In addition, it is also limited by the individual capabilities of the student. These experiences required the student to be proactive and take an interest in the specialty to become an active team member. Therefore, the student's ultimate benefit from these programs could be attributed to his/her comfort as an independent learner to seek information in the research setting.

As research is a longitudinal process and given the time-intensive nature of some projects, it was our experience that a student may need to continue working during his/her "free time" on the project concurrently during subsequent core rotations or classes. The limited time availability could affect the ability of a student to reach the publication or dissemination stage.

It is also recommended that future efforts should be devoted to satisfaction evaluation, not only for the student but the mentor as well. This feedback will provide information that will improve the programs.

CONCLUSION

Outcomes from the two programs were very positive. While the different opportunities and activities within each were varied, programs such as these are very important to encourage participation and instill research skills as scholarly outcomes are mandatory in residency. Beyond training, early engagement in research during medical school could potentially increase interest in academic medicine.

ACKNOWLEDGMENT

We would like to thank Ms. Karen Collins, MPA for her valuable assistance in editing the manuscript.

REFERENCES

[1] Flexner A. *Medical Education in the United States and Canada*. New York, NY: Carnegie Foundation for the Advancement of Teaching; 1910.

[2] Atluru A, Wadhwani A, Maurer K, et al. *Research in medical education: a primer for medical students.* https://www.aamc.org/download/429856/data/mededresearchprimer.pdf. Accessed March 3, 2019.

[3] Pathipati AS, Taleghani N. Research in medical school: a survey evaluating why medical students take research years. *Cureus*. 2016; 8(8). doi:10.7759/cureus.741.

[4] Wickramasinghe DP, Perera CS, Senarathna S, Samarasekera DN. Patterns and trends of medical student research. *BMC Med Educ*. 2013;13(1):175. doi: 10.1186/1472-6920-13-175.

[5] Amgad M, Tsui MMK, Liptrott SJ, Shash E. Medical student research: an integrated mixed-methods systematic review and meta-analysis. *PLoS One*. 2015;10(6). doi:10.1371/journal.pone.0127470.

[6] Association of American Medical Colleges. *The Core Entrustable Professional Activities (EPAs) for Entering Residency.* https://www.aamc.org/initiatives/coreepas/. Accessed April 30, 2019.

[7] Association of American Medical Colleges. *Test Scores and Experiences of First-year Residents, by Specialty.* https://www.aamc.org/data/493918/report-on-residents-2018-b1table.html. Accessed May 5, 2019.

[8] Accreditation Council for Graduate Medical Education (ACGME). *Clinical Learning Environment Review (CLER).* https://www.acgme.org/What-We-Do/Initiatives/Clinical-Learning-Environment-Review-CLER. Accessed April 30, 2019.

[9] Laskowitz DT, Drucker RP, Parsonnet J, Cross PC, Gesundheit N. Engaging students in dedicated research and scholarship during medical school: the long-term experiences at Duke and Stanford. *Acad Med.* 2010;85(3):419-428. doi:10.1097/acm.0b013e3181ccc77a.

[10] Association of American Medical Colleges. *Medical Student Research Requirement.* http://www.aamc.org/initiatives/cir/427194/26.html. Accessed May 7, 2019.

[11] *National Institute of General Medical Sciences: Medical Scientist Training Program.* https://www.nigms.nih.gov/Training/InstPredoc/Pages/PredocOverview-MSTP.aspx. Accessed May 5, 2019.

[12] Brannan, GD. Growing research among osteopathic residents and medical students: a consortium-based research education continuum model. *J Am Osteopath Assoc.* 2016;116(5): 310-315. doi: 10.7556/jaoa.2016.061.

[13] Zemlo TR, Garrison HH, Partridge NC, Ley TJ. The physician-scientist: career issues and challenges at the year 2000. *FASEB J.* 2000;14(2):221-230. doi:10.1096/fasebj.14.2.221.

[14] Havnaer AG, Chen AJ, Greenberg PB. Scholarly concentration programs and medical student research productivity: a systematic review. *Perspect Med Educ.* 2017;6(4): 216-226. doi: 10.1007/s40037-017-0328-2.

[15] Bonilla-Velez J, Small M, Urrutia R, Lomberk G. The enduring value of research in medical education. *Int J Med Stud.* 2017;5(1):37-44. http://www.ijms.info/index.php/IJMS/article/view/168.

[16] Stone C, Dogbey GY, Klenzak S, Van Fossen K, Tan B, Brannan GD. Contemporary global perspectives of medical students on research

during undergraduate medical education: a systematic literature review. *Med Educ Online.* 2018;23(1):1537430. doi: 10.1080/10872981.2018.1537430.

[17] Guelich JM, Singer BH, Castro MC, Rosenberg LE. A gender gap in the next generation of physician-scientists: medical student interest and participation in research. *J Investig Med.* 2002;50(6):412-418. doi:10.1097/00042871-200211010-00024.

[18] Jacobs CD, Cross PC. The value of medical student research: the experience at Stanford University School of Medicine. *Med Educ.* 1995;29(5):342-346. doi:10.1111/j.1365-2923.1995.tb00023.x.

[19] Green EP, Borkan JM, Pross SH, Adler SR, Nothnagle M, Parsonnet J, Gruppuso PA. Encouraging scholarship: medical school programs to promote student inquiry beyond the traditional medical curriculum. *Acad Med.* 2010;85(3):409-18 doi:10.1097/ACM.0b013e3181cd3e00.

[20] Williams R, Holaday L, Lamba S, Soto-Greene M, Sánchez JP. Introducing trainees to medical education activities and opportunities for educational scholarship. *MedEdPORTAL.* 2017 Mar 16;13:10554. doi: 10.15766/mep_2374-8265.10554.

[21] Gotterer GS, O'Day D, Miller BM. The Emphasis program: a scholarly concentrations program at Vanderbilt University School of Medicine. *Acad Med.* 2010;85(11):1717-24. doi:10.1097/ACM.0b013e3181e7771b.

*Reviewed by:*Jay Shubrook, DO, Professor, Touro University College of Osteopathic Medicine, Vallejo, CA, US.

Chapter 3

LEADERSHIP DEVELOPMENT PROGRAMS IN UNDERGRADUATE MEDICAL EDUCATION: UNDERSTANDING THE NEED, BEST PRACTICES AND CHALLENGES

Sumita Sethi[*]
Department of Ophthalmology, BPS GMC for Women,
Sonepat, Haryana, India

ABSTRACT

Medical education, at undergraduate level, has traditionally focused on diagnosis and management of various diseases, with little or no emphasis on team work and leadership necessary to achieve safe and highest quality healthcare. In the modern era, experts and organizations are accepting the need of leadership capabilities in physicians to optimally manage and address the real-life challenges in the rapidly challenging and complex healthcare system. It is important that our young physicians are introduced to their leadership roles in the context of their medical training

---

[*] Corresponding Author's Email: sumitadrss@rrediffmail.com.

and undergraduate medical education provides an ideal setting to lay the foundation of leadership. In contrast to popular belief that 'leaders are born and cannot be made', it has been now established that leadership is made up of a series of definable skills that can be well taught and learnt by dedicated leadership development programs. Despite understanding the undisputed importance of training of leadership skills to medical graduates, most of the medical schools lack formal leadership programs. The chapter discusses the rationale for developing physician-leaders; reviews the need of incorporating leadership development programs in medical curriculum; the best practices of formulating such programs and the expected challenges.

INTRODUCTION

"Leaders wonder about everything, want to learn as much as they can, are willing to take risks, experiment, try new things. They do not worry about failure but embrace errors, knowing they will learn from them."
--Warren G. Bennis
(In: *The Essential Bennis; Essays on Leadership*)

There are many definitions for leaders and managers in literature but most of the researchers agree that *'leaders'* motivate, inspire, and align strategy to establish direction for individuals and the systems in which they work; *'managers'* are process driven and use problem solving to direct individuals and resources to achieve goals already established by leadership [1, 2]. Vroom and Jago, famous in the field of leadership, defined 'leadership' as a process of motivating people to work together collaboratively to accomplish great things [3]. The terms 'leader' and 'manager' are sometimes used interchangeably, but in healthcare they tend to describe different approaches to how change can be achieved [1]. The real challenge is to combine strong leadership and strong management and use each to balance the other [4].

An important threat facing the world today is the lack of effective leadership of our human institutions [5]. The council for advancement of standards in higher education recommends that leadership programs are needed to address advanced student competencies in the foundations of leadership, personal and interpersonal development and development of organizations and systems [6]. Weisbord stated that organizational development, which works well in business models, does not work well in healthcare because of various reasons [7]. The author explained that as part of 'content' of their medical training, health professionals learn rigorous scientific discipline; the 'process' of which inculcates value for personal achievement and importance of improving one's own performance rather than that of institution. The 'science based professional work' thus differs markedly from 'product based organizational work.' The consequences of this lack of effective leadership is evident in health organizations and medical schools [8-9].

Literature review provides evidence of a strong relationship between lack of medical leadership qualities and poor communication and improper health care [10-12]. In the 1990s various researchers and authors argued for improvement in doctor leadership in the delivery of healthcare [13-16]. As per the 1999 Institute of Medicine (IOM) report 'To Err is human', a very high rate of preventable medical error is associated with dysfunctional teamwork or failed communication [17]. It has also been accepted that to ensure high quality patient care and to address the real-life challenges in the rapidly changing and complex health care system, the health organizations and medical schools need competent and effective medical professionals; doctors who have an overall vision and aptitudes that span a variety of process rather than just knowledge of medical procedures [18].

If tomorrow's doctors are expected to be engaged in leadership and management, it is necessary to educate today's medical students. The medical schools have responsibility to make the students develop leadership and management skills so that they can understand multi professional team working [1, 21-22]. Interestingly, the need of leadership skill training as part of their undergraduate curriculum has been appreciated by students themselves. In a study of students' opinion towards leadership and management in undergraduate curriculum, 85% of students thought that they should be taught leadership, teamwork, communication and quality improvement skills [23].

Various accreditation agencies and professional organizations have also accepted need of leadership training in the medical curriculum. The Accreditation council for graduate medical education (ACGME) has accepted ''working effectively as a member or leader of a healthcare team or professional group" as an integral part for all residency programs [24]. The Association of American Medical Colleges (AAMC) has called for ''focus on organizational leadership in the new era of healthcare" [25-26]. The Royal College of Physicians and Surgeons of Canada's CanMEDs physician competency framework includes 'manager' as one of the essential roles [27]. In 2005, report of Royal College of Physicians 'Doctors in Society' argued that 'the competency skills of leadership need to be incorporated into doctors' training so as to support professionalism" [28]. In the United Kingdom, demonstration of competency in the Medical leader Competency framework (MLCF) domains is necessary for satisfactory completion of Annual Review of Competence Progression (ARCP) required for gaining accreditation [29-30]. In the new Competency based curriculum of the Medical Council of India, 'leader' has been recognized as one of the five major roles for the Indian Medical Graduate [31]. A review by Ladhani Z et al. identified leadership and management as amongst the key competencies for undergraduate community-based education for health professionals [32].

Though effective leadership development programs are well-established characteristics of world's most successful organizations, health care organizations have generally lagged behind in implementing such programs; and leadership skills including team-building, conflict management, communication skills are not specifically addressed in most the medical school curricula. Stroller JM commented that it is paradoxical that although teamwork is critical in achieving the highest quality in healthcare, physicians are not trained to be team members or team leaders; instead the traditional physician training is to create 'heroic lone healers' [19,20]. The challenges in healthcare underscore the need to develop healthcare leaders. It is time to think and analyze how the students and physicians are trained in our system and how to teach and cultivate in our medical curriculum to create 'physician-leaders' of tomorrow.

BEST PRACTICES IN FORMULATING STUDENT LEADERSHIP PROGRAMS

"Successful corporations don't wait for leaders to come along. They actively seek out people with leadership potential and expose them to career experiences designed to develop that potential."
--- Kotter [4]

Developing and designing leadership programs for health care institutions, targeting specially the undergraduate students, is challenging; a few questions need to be addressed as pre-requisite for designing such programs.

1. How to define effective leadership in healthcare?
2. Which guiding principles help in describing leadership behavior in different circumstances in healthcare (some of which may be critical)?
3. Are the models of leadership applicable to healthcare as well?
4. Which competencies characterize a physician leader?
5. What features (Instructional methodology, evaluation methods etc.) are ideal to be included in the program?

This section tries to answer these questions in three sections; the first section deals with the various leadership theories and models and how they apply to healthcare; the second section deals with the various leadership competencies and frameworks; and the third section analyze the specific instructional methods used for teaching leadership skills. A cognizance of these factors is the first step towards execution of student leadership programs.

Leadership Models and Guiding Principles

Initially, it was believed that leadership traits are inborn and natural leadership ability is a pre-requisite for developing leaders. Kotter in 1990 argued that leadership is made up of a series of definable skills that can be taught and learnt by dedicated leadership development programs and that all professionals can develop their own ability to lead others [4]. Despite acceptance of this fact, a qualitative study on leadership in healthcare in 2006 concluded that health care leadership development lagged 10-15 years behind leadership development in other industries [33]. Various factors accounted for this, one of which was the lack of a specific model of leadership for healthcare.

Many leadership models have been described in literature; these models define leadership, describe leadership behavior and paths of development of leadership [1, 25, 34]. All these models include the critical components of leadership like integrity, setting vision, inspiring others etc. and each one promotes different ways for how execution of the plan is accomplished. However, every model has its own strategies and goals, understanding of which can help to identify the model that that can best lead to reforms desired. To develop effective leadership skills in healthcare, there is need to identify the models that fit healthcare industry. This section describes the most accepted leadership theories in literature and their relevance to medical education. Some models may work in one particular situation and some may be less useful in other situations.

1. *Transactional leadership:* In this form of leadership, relationships are seen in terms of what the leaders can offer to subordinate and vice-versa [34, 35]. This model, based on systems of reinforcements/awards and punishment/disciplinary action, used to be the most prevalent leadership model in healthcare. However, in contrast to the intrinsic motivation of healthcare providers to 'improve life of others', this model relies on extrinsic motivation of the employee to 'work for his personal interest' [36]. When applied to healthcare, this model has certain shortcomings; firstly, failure to

build trust between a leader and a follower which is an essential part of doctor patient relationship and secondly, failure to take into account ethical and moral obligations of health care providers.

2. *Transformational leadership:* The theory of transformational leadership focuses on stimulating others in the organization to transcend their self-interest to reach higher-order organizational goals [34, 37-39]. This model emphasizes on motivation of group members to raise their awareness of the importance of idealized goals and values. This is then used to address higher-order needs through role modeling, thus providing leadership tailored to enable people to see the alignment of their own personal and professional goals with those of the organization to effect positive change. Bass in 1996, described the four 'I's of transformational leadership; idealized influence (charismatic nature of the leader that makes the followers believe that the leader is worthy of the followers' attention), inspirational motivation (ability of the leader to motivate and inspire other to join in the task), intellectual stimulation (ability of the leader to inspire others to create innovative solutions for the task) and individualized consideration (ability of the leader to address each follower's doubt with a new mission) [37,38,40]. Applied to healthcare, the 'central' role of the transformational leader's vision may inhibit its ability to effect change in health needs; treatment of the patient needs to be individualized and cannot conform to single vision of the transformational leader [40].

3. *Adaptive leadership:* This form of leadership enables a group to overcome challenges created by a change. An adaptive challenge occurs when core beliefs/values lead to failure and a solution to an adaptive challenge involve new behavior, values, roles and approaches to work [39, 40]. Though widely recommended for use in healthcare in clinical settings, its use is limited to a few conditions only, like adaptive challenge when the patient is confronting a high-risk illness [40, 42]. However, it has been accepted that teamwork in healthcare setting requires more decisive action than adaptive leadership allows [40].

4. *Situational leadership:* This model explains how a leader behaves depending on the situation. Hersey and Blanchard in 1993 suggested that situational leaders shift flexibly amongst four behaviors; directing, coaching, supporting and delegating in response to readiness of the follower [43]. If the followers are less capable or lack confidence, a directing or coaching approach is appropriate. However, as capability and confidence increases, leaders can be shifted to more supporting or delegating approach. In medical education, the situational leadership model can be useful for the leaders in appreciating the need for flexibility in their leadership of individuals, committee or teams [40].

5. *Authentic leadership:* As the name indicates, this type of leadership extends from authenticity of the leader to encompass authentic relations with followers [44]. The hallmarks of authentic leaders are knowledge of one's self, ability to self-express beliefs and alignment of concordant goals with those beliefs [34, 46]. This type of leadership is important for students because it focuses on self-awareness that can be developed regardless of positional status and emphasizes the ability to monitor and self-evaluate behavior and emotional reactions [46]. Therefore, authentic leaders are capable to evaluate and use more effective strategies in complex situations.

6. *Servant leadership:* The term apparently came out from Hermann Hesse's *Journey to the East;* and the model first articulated by Greenleaf, refers to response to individuals who are chosen as leaders because they are proven and trusted as servants [47]. The theory proposes that a leader's influence derives from serving the needs of others; characteristic behaviors of servant leadership include listening, empathizing, accepting stewardship and developing others' potential [47, 48]. Servant leadership tends to build trust between healthcare providers and patients and is ethically the soundest form of leadership. However, it may not fit in situations with urgency, like operating room emergency since it may lack the speed needed in such circumstances [40].

At the first instance, the theories may not seem relevant to development of leadership programs in medical education; however, exploring leadership theories and how they relate to professional role of the physician is an essential step towards development of effective leadership skills. Depending on the situation, the models will vary and an effective leader may exhibit a blend of leadership models.

Leadership Competencies and Frameworks

Leadership frameworks consists of competencies which describe the specific knowledge, skills, principles and behavior that contribute to a good performance of learners. In the absence of a dedicated healthcare leadership model, initially business leadership models were being used as foundation to teach leadership skills in medical schools. Based on a systematic review of research in business practices, Wagner et al. in 2011 identified over one hundred seven specific competencies which were then categorized to obtain five major categories; these included self-management, leading others, task management, innovation and social responsibility [49]. Though well-accepted in business practice, it was not yet established whether these types of competencies are relevant to medical education. Violato and Cawthorpe, in a systematic review, identified the various key competencies for teachers, researchers and leaders in medical education; these included medical education expert, educational leadership, curriculum designer, teacher, educational researcher and scholar and learner assessor [50]. Stroller JK had an interesting point of view that though all the frameworks are different in taxonomy and parlance, all of these converge like good statistical models on certain core leadership competencies, similar to those articulated by Kouzes and Posner in their five 'leadership commitments' [20, 51]. According to the authors, great leaders must ''challenge the process, inspire a shared vision, enable others to act, model the way and encourage the heart" [20].

With time, leadership competencies for healthcare started receiving much attention and it was increasingly been accepted by researchers that empirical work was required in medical education leadership [19, 52, 53].

Citaku F et al. in a landmark study, identified social responsibility, innovation, self-management, task management and justice orientation as the perceived competencies for effective leadership in medical education [53]. In this study, some very contrasting differences were observed from the business model by Wagner et al. Firstly, medical education leaders identified social responsibility as the most dominant competency, in contrast to model by Wagner et al. where it was the least important. The authors emphasized that the difference is likely due to emphasis on collaboration and interdisciplinary practice in the health profession, in contrast to competition and independence within business. Another major difference was identification of justice orientation competency which was not part of Wagner et al. model. The authors explained that maintaining safety, following laws and regulations and monitoring progress, as indicated by justice orientation, are critical to medical teaching. In the study, Innovation referred to creative approaches based on sound principles and human resources; Self-management involved setting and achieving goals despite barriers and task management involved planning and efficacy. The authors emphasized that all these competencies are important to provide leadership to health professionals and for managing threats to human health [53].

Taylor et al. proposed four general competencies deemed needed by effective physician-leaders; knowledge, emotional intelligence, vision, and selfless dedication to the organization [54]. Their findings validated results of other studies regarding leadership competencies in specific context of healthcare; the themes in their study closely resembled those by Kouzes and Posner as five key leadership challenges [51]. In another systematic review, Stoller suggested six domains of competencies for effective physician-leadership; these include technical skills and knowledge (regarding operational, financial, and information systems, human resources, and strategic planning); industry knowledge (e.g., regarding clinical processes, regulation, and healthcare trends); problem-solving skills; emotional intelligence; communication, and finally a commitment to lifelong learning [55]. Ladhani L et al. had an interesting analysis which indicated that the recommended leadership competencies across the globe tend to cluster in three domains; understanding self, leading and managing and understanding healthcare system [56].

Chen TY in his study pointed out that various leadership curricula in undergraduate medical education focus on a wide range of competencies, but they are often not consistent with existing leadership competency framework [1]. Allison MB Webb et al. did an extensive review of articles describing curricula with interventions leadership skills to teach medical students [22]. They concluded Medical Leadership Competency Framework (MLCF) as the most comprehensive and detailed model for leadership education in medicine. The MLCF, developed by the United Kingdom National Health Service (UK NHS) institute for innovation and improvement and academy of Medical Royal Colleges, gives an outline of leadership competencies expected of a practicing clinician [57]. There are five domains of leadership and within each domain, there are four elements and each of the four elements are further divided into four competency outcomes. The five domains are demonstrating personal qualities, working with others, managing services, improving services and setting direction. The authors emphasized that aligning leadership curricula with competency models such as MLCF would create opportunities to standardize evaluation of outcomes, thus leading to better measurement of student competency and better understanding of the best practices [22].

While MLCF is a dedicated framework developed to direct leadership training for medical students and physicians, there are a few others in literature which are accepted as health care leadership models. The Duke Healthcare Model, proposed by Charles William Hargett et al. features the central core principle of patient centredness which is surrounded by five overlapping core competencies [58]. The authors utilized concept mapping approach to derive, prioritize and thematically structure the fundamental competencies of leadership in medicine to create a model specific to the needs of learning in healthcare leadership. Emotional intelligence was recognized as core competency that holds all other competency together and is positioned as keystone in the model; critical thinking and teamwork were positioned as the fundamental core competencies. Another popular model is that of the National Center for health care leadership model (NCHL) which has three domains – transformation, execution and people; and these are further defined by twenty-six leadership competencies such as analytical thinking, interpersonal understanding etc [59]. Stroller JK et al. defined emotional intelligence (EI) as the ability to understand and manage oneself; to understand others and manage relationships; and emphasized that amongst the competencies needed by leaders, EI is the one that has been shown to differentiate between great and average leaders [60]. The authors recommended teaching specific components of EI like teambuilding, empathy, and negotiation as part of the medical training. Literature suggests EI to be a critical leadership competency for healthcare providers [59-61].

The first step for a well-designed and well-evaluated program is deciding the framework and identifying the respective competencies and objectives in advance and thereafter ensuring their alignment to the teaching learning methods.

Teaching Learning Format and Instructional Methodology

One of the unique characteristics of leadership studies is that it transcends the disciplines and prepares students for all professionals. Before deciding which teaching learning format and instructional methodology is appropriate for development of leadership in healthcare, it is important to know the background how the various teaching learning methodologies have evolved over time. This section first gives an insight into how the teaching methodology of leadership evolved and then describes how they were applied to healthcare leadership and thereafter analyses literature about the common and accepted methods for student leadership programs.

Conger and his research team in 1992 were the first to categorize leadership training format into four key approaches; Personal growth, Conceptual, Feedback and Skill building [62]. Several years later, Allen and Hartman in 2008 and later in 2009, built upon Conger's work and created one of the most comprehensive list of leadership development teaching methods found in literature [63-65]. Nearly simultaneously, a very interesting and important concept of signature pedagogies in teaching of leadership skills was introduced by Shulman in 2005; he identified effective signature pedagogies as the forms of instruction that incorporate active student participation, make students feel deeply engaged and promote a learning environment where students visible [66]. According to his description, signature pedagogies are those teaching methods which first come to a faculty's mind when he is asked to identify the most dominant instructional strategies used to teach a specific discipline. Interestingly, though Shulman's model was being applied to many other disciplines, there was no literature which discussed signature pedagogies in the leadership discipline.

Making use of Schulman's philosophy and instructional strategies offered by Allen and Hartman, Jenkins DM did an exhaustive review to explore the instructional strategies most frequently used by leadership educators and to identify signature pedagogies in undergraduate leadership education [67]. Similar to four approach models of leadership development by Conger and Allen and Hartman, the authors grouped the instructional strategies into four groups; personal growth, conceptual understanding, feedback and skill building. The study focused on twenty-four instructional strategies including twelve of Allen and Hartman and concluded that class discussion, whether in form of true class discussion or interactive lecture and discussion are used most frequently, thus identifying it as the signature pedagogy for leadership education; other being projects and presentation, self-assessment and critical reflections. Henal Shah et al. in a recent paper analyzed whether the teaching learning methods identified by Jenkins were generalizable to a global leadership curriculum for mid-career health professional's faculty as well [68]. It was an interesting conclusion that similar to Jenkin's report, reflection and interactive discussion were two very frequently used teaching learning methods for health professionals as well.

Warren Oliver et al. in their review paper described the most frequently used leadership development methodologies in various leadership programs [69]. The first described methodology was *'Mentoring'* which is defined as offline help by one person to another in making significant transitions in knowledge, work, and thinking [69, 70]. Though associated with multiple benefits to both mentors and mentees, the authors strongly advocate that it is beneficial for any aspiring medical leader to establish a mentoring relationship for personal and professional development. However, if mentoring is to be used as a tool for leadership development, one must be aware of its potential limitations and consider a more formalized process to establish mentor mentee pairings [71]. The second method described is that of *'Coaching'*; this is a relatively short-term process and is aimed at performance enhancement in a specific area [69, 72]. What happens in the coaching process that can support leadership development is not known in literature but it is accepted as a method for development of leadership for more senior doctors when appointed to leadership roles. The third method described is *'Action learning'* which is based on the notion that joint problem solving of issues that arise in work-place, during real life projects can be used to develop leadership knowledge, skills and attitude [69]. The aim of this method is not to give advice but to help and empower the individual to reach their own conclusions. The fourth methodology is *'Networking'* which according to authors play an important part in leadership development and when successful, it may be sustained over a longer period than coaching and mentoring [69]. Networking tends to involve creation of interdependent, often mutually beneficial relationships and it occurs in two distinct ways; peer networking and networking with senior leaders. The last methodology described is that of *'Experiential learning'* which involves real challenge in form of 'stretch assignments' that tend to offer important developmental opportunities, requiring the individual to work outside their comfort zone and also learn new skills to achieve the desired outcomes. Experiential learning is one of the most appreciated methodology in literature and there is evidence of learners' satisfaction with this type of leaning opportunities which empower them to apply leadership skills [25, 69, 73-77].

There is strong evidence that training leadership skills in isolation from the specialized context is to be avoided and it is important to take into account explicitly of clinical requirements and cooperation of medical teams [53]. Various curricular and extracurricular activities have been described in literature for teaching of leadership skills [78-88]. Renae Chesnut et al.

assessed the effectiveness of the student Leadership Development Series (SLDS), an academic year long, co-curricular approach, to develop leadership skills in pharmacy students [84]. The program provided the students with a foundation curriculum that used co-curricular activities including guest speakers and students' own research presented in a poster session. Jorge ML et al. described an optional curricular activity that was designed to introduce students to the hospital community and to provide guidance in practical and management activities in a quality control laboratory [87]. The purpose was to put students in a position where they need to apply their knowledge in day to day activities that make them develop critical analysis, resolve problems and manage people. A simulation-based curriculum was described by Arna Banerjee et al. to introduce key teamwork principles as part of the foundation course for beginning medical students [88]. The authors emphasized that simulation fulfills the basic human need 'to learn with active participation'; also allowing simultaneously reflection on the experience and facilitates incorporation of behavioral changes into personal practice.

Mark T. O. Connell analyzed eight leadership and teamwork curricular projects from US medical schools and concluded that the most common identified curricular approach to teach leadership and teamwork was clinical case rounds to specifically demonstrate the roles, responsibilities and interactions among physicians and other members of multidisciplinary team [89]. Clinical rotations were also identified as a great opportunity for leadership development by 62% of undergraduate students in a study by Varkey P et al. [83]. In a recent systematic review on leadership training in graduate medical education, Sadowski B et al. did an exhaustive analysis of published literature in graduate leadership curricula; multiple teaching modalities were used and small group teaching, mentoring, coaching and project work were identified as the most effective approaches based on available resources and learner preference. Project learning was identified as a powerful motivational tool that enhanced accountability allowing participants to apply leadership skills [21].

Literature shows that there are two different approaches to offer leadership education to students; first a cohesive leadership and medical degree program which would require additional year of training; secondly, a longitudinal integrated program with opportunity to develop leadership [21]. A four-year integrated curriculum, to engage with leadership roles starting early in the pre-clinical stages of training was described by Clyne B at al.; the sessions were designed to be goal oriented, related to prior experience, practical and interactive and teaching methods were intended to encourage teamwork and higher-order thinking skills making use of techniques like debate, expert panels, simulators, public speaking, case analysis and reflective writing. A critical component of the program was an experiential learning activity which allowed students to apply learning activity that allowed students to apply lessons learned in class to their leadership development [25].

A flexible credit leadership elective course, developed and taught by graduate students that used a wide variety of texts and scholarly publications to provide students with a range of materials discussing leadership topics was described by Patterson BJ et al. [73]. This was based on Kneflekamp and Widick's seminal development instruction model which describes four elements to deliver educational experiences that meet the needs of student learners (framework, diversity, experiential learning and personalism) [73, 90]. The authors emphasized use of authentic leadership by using reflective contemplation to drive their own learning which enables students to develop lifelong leadership development skills from chosen opportunities and life experiences.

THE CHALLENGES

"Leaders are perpetual learners."
--- Warren G. Bennis (in *Leaders: The Strategies for Taking Charge*)

Developing and designing effective systems for developing specific leadership competencies and evaluating their impact is in itself a challenging task. It is important that students' individual learning preferences are accommodated while planning such courses [69]. This allows a tailored approach for leadership programs, thus enhancing self-awareness of participants and allowing them to monitor their own progress. Though there is clear evidence in literature for the competencies and domains for leadership programs to be adhered to a standardized framework; it is important that the institute develops their own leadership curriculum. Even widely supported models like MLCF have frequently been criticized for laying responsibility on an individual without any regard for the context and environment in which they operate [91].

Literature indicates that there is need to focus on leadership development for all healthcare professionals, starting early and continuing throughout their career [69]. However, it is important to decide the optimum time for introducing such programs to be most effective. Given the present-day undergraduate curriculum, there is little room for adding more content to it. It has been accepted that longitudinal or serial sessions are preferred over a single event; there is need to identify ways through which leadership curriculum is integrated longitudinally in the preexisting curriculum.

Leadership needs to be developed at all levels of health organizations. It is important that in the process of developing physician leaders of tomorrow, today's health professionals and educators are also involved; professional development activities targeting leadership skills for faculty members will help them develop as role models for the students. Another important consideration is that of resources; to allow the physicians to lead across professional boundaries and become efficient leaders, most of the leadership programs will also need certain non-technical skills; developing these attributes will require dedicated resources and specific instructional methodology [69]. While planning the leadership development programs, it is important that instructional methods are identified based on desired outcomes and available resources and opportunities and resources are provided for development of technical as well as non-technical skills.

Another major challenge is evaluation of such programs; there are contrasting views regarding assessment of leadership skills; some argue that assessment would reduce interest and would constitute another opportunity for them to just pass or fail or to score; few others argue that without assessment, there would be no measurable outcomes to evaluate learning and that there should be minimum standards that the student need to achieve [23]. Various methods have been described in literature for evaluation of leadership programs; however, in most of the studies, the criteria of success represent the simplest evaluation step in Kirkpatrick model [21, 52]. Surveys and knowledge assessments are easy to obtain and are useful criteria in program feedback but fail to capture the full effectiveness of leadership programs [21]. Comprehensive data like multisource feedback could better define higher Kirkpatrick levels; also leadership skills rating scales, applied to students and compared before and after completing the leadership development program, can be used to assess students learning from the program [92]. Feedback, reflections, written short reports of observed scenario or real practice, critical appraisal, verbal assessments, monthly implementation forms, poster presentation, creation of students' leadership platform, travel scholarship reflection etc. have all been suggested to be useful [21]. It is thus important that evaluation is planned in such a way that higher levels of Kirkpatrick model are targeted. Leadership is an ongoing process and thus it is desirable to have longitudinal follow-ups to understand how the physician has evaluated as a leader.

CONCLUSION AND FUTURE DIRECTIONS

'There is nothing in a physician's training that qualifies him to be a leader.'
--- Larry Mathis (in *Lessons in Leadership*)

In most of the medical schools, students take part in various activities with peers, patients, teachers and multidisciplinary teams but their role in most of the practical activities is limited to observation and no demands are made to them to take responsibility of their actions. However, when it comes to real life scenario, they are accountable for their professional activities and have to assume leadership roles in various capacities. There is thus an apparent gap between their 'training as students' and 'expectations as physician leaders'; this inattention to development of leadership skills are amongst a few factors which provide the rationale for dedicated leadership development programs. Well-designed and well-evaluated leadership development programs targeting the medical students, more specifically the undergraduates, aims to fulfill these gaps. Through various leadership related activities, these programs tend to ensure that doctors, at any stage of their medical training, attain an agreed set of leadership competencies thus preparing them for their role as future physician leaders and for developing their self-efficacy as leaders.

Medical schools should develop their own leadership curricula and identify the key competencies and skills they want to focus. It is of the utmost importance to understand which leadership skills a physician needs and for this research is to be targeted to requirement analysis at different hierarchical levels. Leadership development is an ongoing process, health care institutions must provide opportunities and resources for health professionals to develop as leaders at all levels [93]. Simultaneously high-quality research is needed to study evaluation methods for such programs. The evaluation methods should target pre and post training performance of participants and the transfer of content to everyday clinical practice; this will be an indicator of the effectiveness and value of the program. In the future, there is need and opportunity to focus on outcomes at higher level of Kirkpatrik evaluation scale and qualitative approach to understand the complexity of leadership development and its significance from perspectives of students. There is need for collaboration at all levels towards creating a culture of leadership to improve design and delivery of medical education and healthcare.

ACKNOWLEDGMENTS

As part of fellowship at FAIMER Regional Institute (FRI), GSMC, Mumbai (2019 batch), the author is working on an educational innovation project on leadership development in medical students; the author wants to acknowledge FAIMER faculty at GSMC, Mumbai for providing continuous guidance for the project. During working on the project (unpublished data) and going through literature exhaustively, the author decided to write the chapter so that the concepts can be shared with the scientific community.

REFERENCES

[1] Chen TY. Medical leadership: An important and required competency for medical students. *Ci Ji Yi Xue Za Zhi*. 2018 Apr-Jun;30(2):66-70. doi: 10.4103/tcmj.tcmj_26_18.

[2] Aggarwal R, Swanwick T. Clinical leadership development in postgraduate medical education and training: policy, strategy, and delivery in the UK National Health Service. *J Healthc Leadersh*. 2015 Nov 17;7:109-122. doi: 10.2147/JHL.S69330.

[3] Vroom VH, Jago AG. The role of the situation in leadership. *Am Psychol*. 2007 Jan;62(1):17-24; discussion 43-7.

[4] Kotter JP. What leaders really do. *Harv Bus Rev*. 1990 May-Jun;68(3):103-11.

[5] Bennis W. The challenges of leadership in the modern world: introduction to the special issue. *Am Psychol*. 2007 Jan;62(1):2-5; discussion 43-7.

[6] Council for the advancement of standards in higher education (CAS). *CAS Professional Standards for Higher Education*, 7th ed. Washington, DC:CAS;2009.

[7] Weisbord MR. Why organization development hasn't worked (so far) in medical centers. *Health Care Manage Rev*. 1976 Spring;1(2):17-28.

[8] Bisbee DC. Looking for leaders: current practices in leadership identification in higher education. *Planning and Changing* 2007;38:77-78.

[9] Zaccaro SJ. Trait-based perspectives of leadership. *Am Psychol*. 2007 Jan;62(1):6-16; discussion 43-7.

[10] Hamilton P, Spurgeon P, Clark J, Dent J, and Armit K. Engaging Doctors: Can doctors influence organizational performance? *NHS Institute for Innovation and Improvement Coventry*, 2008.

[11] Pham JC, Aswani MS, Rosen M, Lee H, Huddle M, Weeks K, Pronovost PJ. Reducing medical errors and adverse events. *Annu Rev Med.* 2012;63:447-63. doi: 10.1146/annurev-med-061410-121352.
[12] Mazzocco K, Petitti DB, Fong KT, Bonacum D, Brookey J, Graham S, Lasky RE, Sexton JB, Thomas EJ. Surgical team behaviors and patient outcomes. *Am J Surg.* 2009 May;197(5):678-85. doi: 10.1016/j.amjsurg.2008.03.002
[13] Keen J, Buxton M, Packwood T. Doctors and resource management: incentives and goodwill. *Health Policy* 1993;24:71-82.
[14] Chantler C. Reinventing doctors. Will move doctors from this winter of discontent to a position of leadership. *BMJ* 1998;317:1670-1671.
[15] Chantler C. Interdisciplinary relationships. *J R Soc Med* 1998;91:317-18.
[16] Chantler C. The role and education of doctors in the delivery of health care. *Lancet* 1999;353:1178-81.
[17] Kohn LT, Corrigan JM, Donaldson MS, Institute of Medicine (U.S.), Committee on Quality of Healthcare in America. *To err is human: Building a safer health system.* Washington: National Academy Press; 2000. p. 311.
[18] Veronesi G, Kirkpatrick I, Vallascas F. Clinicians on the board: what difference does it make? *Soc Sci Med.* 2013 Jan;77:147-55. doi: 10.1016/j.socscimed.2012.11.019.
[19] Stoller JK. Developing physician-leaders: a call to action. *J Gen Intern Med.* 2009 Jul;24(7):876-8. doi: 10.1007/s11606-009-1007.
[20] Stoller JK. Developing Physician Leaders: A Perspective on Rationale, Current Experience, and Needs. *Chest.* 2018 Jul;154(1):16-20. doi:10.1016/j.chest.2017.12.014.
[21] Sadowski B, Cantrell S, Barelski A, O'Malley PG, Hartzell JD. Leadership Training in Graduate Medical Education: A Systematic Review. *J Grad Med Educ.* 2018 Apr;10(2):134-148. doi: 10.4300/JGME-D-17-00194.1.
[22] Webb AM, Tsipis NE, McClellan TR, McNeil MJ, Xu M, Doty JP, Taylor DC. A first step toward understanding best practices in leadership training in undergraduate medical education: a

systematic review. *Acad Med.* 2014 Nov;89(11):1563-70. doi: 10.1097/ACM.0000000000000502.

[23] Quince T, Abbas M, Murugesu S, Crawley F, Hyde S, Wood D, Benson J. Leadership and management in the undergraduate medical curriculum: a qualitative study of students' attitudes and opinions at one UK medical school. *BMJ Open.* 2014 Jun 25;4(6):e005353. doi: 10.1136/bmjopen-2014-005353.

[24] Accreditation Council for Graduate Medical Education. *The outcome project.* [Online] 2014 [cited 2019 May 23]. Available from: URL: www.ACGME.org.

[25] Clyne B, Rapoza B, George P. Leadership in Undergraduate Medical Education: Training Future Physician Leaders. *R I Med J* (2013). 2015 Sep 1;98(9):36-40.

[26] Enders T, Conroy I. Washington, D.C: The Association of American Medical Colleges; 2014. *Advancing the academic health system for the future: A report for the AAMC health advisory panel.*

[27] Frank JR. *The CanMEDS 2005 Physician Competency Framework.* Ottawa: The Royal College of Physicians and Surgeons of Canada; 2005. Available from: http://www.royalcollege.ca/portal/page/portal/rc/common/documents/canmeds/resources/publications/framework_full_e.pdf.

[28] *Doctors in Society. Medical Professionalism in a changing world.* London: Royal College of Physicians, 2005.

[29] NHS Institute for Innovation and Improvement. The clinical leadership competency framework. *Coventry*, 2011.

[30] Bethune R, Soo E, Woodhead P, et al. Engaging all doctors in continuous quality improvement: a structured, supported programme for first-year doctors across a training deanery in England. *BMJ Qual Saf* 2013;22:613–17.

[31] Medical Council of India. *Competency based undergraduate curriculum for the Indian Medical Graduate* [online] 2019 [cited 2019 May 29]. Available from https://www.mciindia.org/CMS/wp-content/uploads/2019/01/UG-Curriculum-Vol-I.pdf.

[32] Ladhani Z, Scherpbier AJ, Stevens FJ. Competencies for undergraduate community based education for the health professions: a systematic review. *Med Teach* 2012;39:733–43.

[33] McAleamey AS. Leadership development in healthcare: a qualitative study. *J Organiz Behav.* 2006;27(7):967-982.

[34] J. McKimm, S. J. Lieff. *A practical guide for medical teachers*, Edition: 4, Publisher: Churchill Livingstone/Elsevier, 2013, Editors: John Dent; Ronald M Harden, Chapter: Medical Education Leadership, pp.343-352.

[35] Bass BM: *Transformational leadership*, ed.2, Mahwah, NJ, 1996,Lawrence Erlbaum.

[36] Kreps DM. Intrinsic motivation and extrinsic incentives. *Am Econ Rev.* 1997; 87(2):359-364.

[37] Bass BM, Avolio B*: Improving organizational effectiveness through transformational leadership*, Thousand Oaks, NJ, 1994, Sage.

[38] Xirasagar S, Samuels ME, Stoskopf CH. Physician leadership styles and effectiveness: an empirical study. *Med Care Res Rev.* 2005 Dec;62(6):720-40.

[39] Northouse PG. *Leadership theory and practice.* 3rd edition. Thousand Oaks, CA: Sage; 2004:170-200.

[40] Trastek VF, Hamilton NW, Niles EE. Leadership models in health care - a case for servant leadership. *Mayo Clin Proc.* 2014 Mar;89(3):374-81. doi: 10.1016/j.mayocp.2013.10.012.

[41] Heifetz RA, Laune DL. The work of leadership. *Har Bus Rev.* 1997;75(1):124-134.

[42] Haeusler JM. Medicine needs adaptive leadership. *Physician Exec.* 2010;36(2):12-15.

[43] Hersey P, Blanchard K. *Management of organizational behavior. Utilizing human resources.* 6th ed. Englewood Cliffs: Prentice Hall;1993.

[44] Luthans F, Avolio BJ: Authentic leadership: A positive developmental approach. In Cameron KS, Dutton JE, Quinn RE, editors: *Positive Organizational Scholarship.* San Francisco 2003 Barrett-Koehler, pp24—261.

[45] Avolio BJ. *Leadership development in balance: MADE/Born.* Mahwah, NJ: Lawrence Erlbaum;2005.
[46] Gardner WL, Avolio BJ, Luthans F et al. Can you see the real me? A self based model of authentic leader and follower development. *Leadership Q.* 2005;16(3):343-372.
[47] Greenleaf RK. *Servant Leadership: a journey into the nature of legitimate power and greatness.* New York, NY: Paulist Press; 1977.
[48] Spears LC. Practicing servant leadership. *Leader to Leader.* 2004;34:7-11.
[49] Wagner S, Bapat A, Bennett M, et al. *A Leadership Competency Model.* Central Michigan University, 2011. http://www.chsbs.cmich.edu/leader_model.
[50] Violato C, Cawthorpe D. Core Research Competencies for Scholars and Researchers in Medical Education: an MSc and PhD Program. Research in *Medical Education—Chances and Challenges.* Düsseldorf: German Medical Science GMS Publishing House, 2009;20:22.
[51] Kouzes J, Posner B. *The leadership challenge.* 5th ed. New York: Wiley;2012.
[52] Kiesewetter J, Schmidt-Huber M, Netzel J, Krohn AC, Angstwurm M, Fischer MR. Training of leadership skills in medical education. *GMS Z Med Ausbild.* 2013 Nov 15;30(4):Doc49.
[53] Citaku F, Violato C, Beran T, Donnon T, Hecker K, Cawthorpe D. Leadership competencies for medical education and healthcare professions: population-based study. *BMJ Open.* 2012 Mar 27;2(2):e000812. doi: 10.1136/bmjopen-2012-000812.
[54] Taylor CA, Taylor JC, Stoller JK. Exploring leadership competencies in established and aspiring physician leaders: an interview-based study. *J Gen Intern Med.* 2008;23:748–754.
[55] Stoller JK. Developing physician-leaders: key competencies and available programs. *J Health Adm Educ.* 2008 Fall;25(4):307-28.

[56] Ladhani Z, Shah H, Wells R et al. Global Leadership Model for Health Professions Education – A Case Study of the FAIMER program. *Journal of Leadership Education* 2015;14(4):67-91. DOI: 1012806/VI4/I4/R1.

[57] Academy of Medical Royal Colleges. *Medical Leadership Competency Framework: Enhancing Engagement in Medical Leadership.* 3rd ed. Coventry, UK: NHS Institute for Innovation and Improvement; 2010. https://www.leadershipacademy.nhs.uk/wp-content/uploads/2012/11/NHSLeadership-Leadership-Framework-Medical-Leadership-Competency-Framework-3rd-ed.pdf. Accessed February 7, 2019.

[58] Hargett CW, Doty JP, Hauck JN, Webb AM, Cook SH, Tsipis NE, Neumann JA, Andolsek KM, Taylor DC. Developing a model for effective leadership in healthcare: a concept mapping approach. *J Healthc Leadersh.* 2017 Aug 28;9:69-78. doi: 10.2147/JHL.S141664.

[59] Dine CJ, Kahn JM, Abella BS, Asch DA, Shea JA. Key elements of clinical physician leadership at an academic medical center. *J Grad Med Educ.* 2011 Mar;3(1):31-6. doi: 10.4300/JGME-D-10-00017.1.

[60] Stoller JK, Taylor CA, Farver CF. Emotional intelligence competencies provide a developmental curriculum for medical training. *Med Teach.* 2013;35(3):243-7. doi: 10.3109/0142159X.2012.737964.

[61] Keith SJ, Buckley PF. Leadership experiences and characteristics of chairs of academic departments of psychiatry. *Acad Psychiatry.* 2011 Mar-Apr;35(2):118-21. doi: 10.1176/appi.ap.35.2.118.

[62] Conger, J. (1992*). Learning to lead: The art of transforming managers into leaders.* San Francisco: Jossey-Bass.

[63] Allen, S. J., & Hartman, N. S. (2008a). Leadership development: An exploration of sources of learning. *SAM Advanced Management Journal*, 73(1), 10– 19, 62.

[64] Allen, S. J., & Hartman, N. S. (2008b). Sources of learning: An exploratory study. *Organization Development Journal*, 26(2), 75–87.

[65] Allen, S. J., & Hartman, N. S. (2009). Sources of learning in student leadership development programming. *Journal of Leadership Studies*, 3(3), 6-16.

[66] Shulman, L. S. (2005). Signature pedagogies in the disciplines. *Daedalus,* 134(3), 52-59.

[67] Jenkins DM. Exploring Signature Pedagogies in undergraduate Leadership Education. *Journal of Leadership Education* 2012;11(1):1-27.

[68] Shah H, Ladhani Z, Morahan PS et al. *Global Leadership Model for Health Professions Education Part 2: Teaching/Learning Methods* 2019; 18(12):193-200.

[69] Warren OJ, Carnall R. Medical leadership: why it's important, what is required, and how we develop it. *Postgrad Med J.* 2011 Jan;87(1023):27-32. doi: 10.1136/pgmj.2009.093807.

[70] Clutterbuck D. *Everyone needs a mentor-Fostering talent in your organization.* 4th ed. London: CIPD;2004.

[71] Warren O, Humphris P. The role of mentoring in academic surgery. In: Athanasiou T, Darzi A, Debas HT, eds. *Key points in surgical research.* Berlin:Springer Scientific, 2009.

[72] Flaherty J. *Coaching: Evoking excellence in others.* Boston, MA: Butterworth-Heinemann; 1999.

[73] Patterson BJ, Garza OW, Witry MJ, Chang EH, Letendre DE, Trewet CB. A leadership elective course developed and taught by graduate students. *Am J Pharm Educ.* 2013 Dec 16;77(10):223. doi: 10.5688/ajpe7710223.

[74] Blumenthal DM, Bernard K, Fraser TN, et al. Implementing a pilot leadership course for internal medicine residents: design considerations, participant impressions, and lessons learned. *BMC Med Educ.* 2014;14:257.

[75] Doughty RA, Williams PD, Seashore CN. Chief resident training. Developing leadership skills for future medical leaders. *Am J Dis Child.* 1991;145(6):639–642.

[76] Lee MT, Tse AM, Naguwa GS. Building leadership skills in paediatric residents. *Med Educ.* 2004;38(5):559–560.

[77] Levine SA, Chao SH, Brett B, et al. Chief resident immersion training in the care of older adults: an innovative interspecialty education and leadership intervention. *J Am Geriatr Soc.* 2008;56(6):1140–1145.

[78] Wipf JE, Pinsky LE, Burke W. Turning interns into senior residents: preparing residents for their teaching and leadership roles. *Acad Med.* 1995;70(7):591–596. doi: 10.1097/00001888-199507000-00010.

[79] Levine SA, Chao SH, Brett B, Jackson AH, Burrows AB, Goldman LN, Caruso LB. Chief Resident Immersion Training in the Care of Older Adults: An Innovative Interspecialty Education and Leadership Intervention. *J Am Geriatr Soc.* 2008;56(6):1140–1145. doi: 10.1111/j.1532-5415.2008.01710.

[80] Awad SS, Hayley B, Fagan SP, Berger DH, Brunicardi FC. The impact of a novel resident leadership training curriculum. *Am J Surg.* 2004;188(5):481–484. doi: 10.1016/j.amjsurg.2004.07.024.

[81] Devaul RA, Knight JA, Edwards KA. Leadership training in medical education. *Med Teach.* 1994;16(1):47–51. doi: 10.3109/01421599409108257.

[82] Ayuob NN, Al Sayes FM, El Deek BS. Extracurricular leadership development programme to prepare future Saudi physicians as leaders. *J Pak Med Assoc.* 2016 Jun;66(6):688-93.

[83] Varkey P, Peloquin J, Reed D, Lindor K, Harris I. Leadership curriculum in undergraduate medical education: a study of student and faculty perspectives. *Med Teach.* 2009 Mar;31(3):244-50. doi: 10.1080/01421590802144278.

[84] Chesnut R, Tran-Johnson J. Impact of a student leadership development program. *Am J Pharm Educ.* 2013 Dec 16;77(10):225. doi: 10.5688/ajpe7710225.

[85] Hemmer PR, Karon BS, Hernandez JS, Cuthbert C, Fidler ME, Tazelaar HD. Leadership and management training for residents and fellows: a curriculum for future medical directors. *Arch Pathol Lab Med.* 2007 Apr;131(4):610-4.

[86] Janke KK, Nelson MH, Bzowyckyj AS, Fuentes DG, Rosenberg E, DiCenzo R. Deliberate Integration of Student Leadership

Development in Doctor of Pharmacy Programs. *Am J Pharm Educ.* 2016 Feb 25;80(1):2. doi: 10.5688/ajpe8012.

[87] Jorge ML, Coelho IC, Paraizo MM, Paciornik EF. Leadership, management and teamwork learning through an extra-curricular project for medical students: descriptive study. *Sao Paulo Med J.* 2014;132(5):303-6.

[88] Banerjee A, Slagle JM, Mercaldo ND, Booker R, Miller A, France DJ, Rawn L, Weinger MB. A simulation-based curriculum to introduce key teamwork principles to entering medical students. *BMC Med Educ.* 2016 Nov 16;16(1):295.

[89] O'Connell MT, Pascoe JM. Undergraduate medical education for the 21st century: leadership and teamwork. *Fam Med.* 2004 Jan;36 Suppl:S51-6.

[90] Kneflekamp L, Widick C. Developmental instruction model. In: Evans NJ, Forney DS, Guido-DiBrito F, eds. *Student Developent in College: Theory, Research, and Practice.* San Francisco, CA: Jossey-Bass; 1998:91-98.

[91] Bolden R, Gosling J. Leadership competencies: time to change the tune? *Leadership* 2006;2:147-63.

[92] Australian continuous improvement group, ACIG. *Leadership Skills- How Do You Rate?* [Online] 2000 [cited 2014 May 2]. Available from: URL: http://www.acig.com.au/wp-content/uploads/2011/03/ToolsEffectiveMeetingsLeadershipQuestionnaire.pdf?phpMyAdmin=jdFVqNrw5Z9ZWRTBDv0hu9XJ0na.

[93] Steinert Y, Naismith L, Mann K. Faculty development initiatives designed to promote leadership in medical education. A BEME systematic review: BEME Guide No. 19. *Med Teach.* 2012;34(6):483-503. doi: 10.3109/0142159X.2012.680937.

BIOGRAPHICAL SKETCH

Sumita Sethi

Affiliation:
- Associate Professor Ophthalmology, BPS GMC, Sonepat
- Resource faculty Medical Education Unit BPS GMC, Sonepat
- Additional resource faculty MCI Regional Centre for Faculty Development, Maulana Azad Medical College, New Delhi

Education:
- MBBS, M.S. (Ophthalmology),
- Medical Council of India Advance Course in medical Education (ACME), 2017 batch
- Presently enrolled for Foundation for advancement of International Medical Education and Research (FAIMER) Regional Institute (2019 batch) at GSMC-FAIMER Regional Institute, Mumbai, India

Business Address: BPS GMC for Women, Khanpur, Sonepat, Haryana, India

Research and Professional Experience:
- Sr. Residency (Pediatric Ophthalmology) (December 2004 – December 2007): Chacha Nehru children hospital, Maulana Azad Medical College, New Delhi.
- Sr. Research associateship (pediatric eye oncology) (May 2008 – May 2011): Department of pediatric ophthalmology and oncology, Dr. Rajendra Prasead Centre for ophthalmic sciences, All India Institute of Medical Sciences, New Delhi.

Professional Appointments:
- Assistant Professor (Ophthalmology) (January 2012 – January 2016): BPS Government medical college for women, Khanpur Kalan, Sonepat, Haryana.
- Present Designation (January 2016 till date): Associate professor of Ophthalmology, BPS Government medical college for women, Khanpur Kalan, Sonepat, Haryana.
- Additional resource faculty MCI Regional Centre for Faculty Development, Maulana Azad Medical College, New Delhi (Since May 2019)

Honors:
- *Best Senior research associate award;* Dr. Rajendra Prasad Centre for ophthalmic sciences, All India Institute of Medical Science, 2011.
- *Most popular teacher (Clinical) award, 2015;* National Medicos Organization, Haryana

Publications from the Last 3 Years:
1. Sethi S, Badyal DK. Clinical procedural skills assessment during internship in ophthalmology. *J Adv Med Educ Prof.* 2019 Apr;7(2):56-61. PubMed PMID: 31086797; PubMed Central PMCID: PMC6475030.
2. Sethi S, Siwach A, Dabas R, Verma S. An analysis of macular thickness in amblyopic eyes in rural India by spectral optical coherence tomography. *Oman J Ophthalmol.* 2018 Sep-Dec;11(3):304-305. doi: 10.4103/ojo.OJO_26_2017. PubMed PMID: 30505133; PubMed Central PMCID: PMC6219327.
3. Ganesh S, Gupta R, Sethi S, Gurung C, Mehta R. Myopic Shift After Intraocular Lens Implantation in Children Less Than Two Years of Age. *Nepal J Ophthalmol.* 2018 Jan;10(19):11-15. doi: 10.3126/nepjoph.v10i1.21662. PubMed PMID: 31056571.
4. Ganesh S, Tibrewal S, Yadav A, Sethi S. Anomalous Lateral Rectus Muscle Band in a Case of Duane Retraction Syndrome. *Strabismus.*

2017 Dec;25(4):191-194. doi: 10.1080/09273972.2017.1392989. Epub 2017 Nov 14. PubMed PMID: 29135308.
5. Reddy VS, Sethi S, Agrawal P, Gupta N, Garg R. Ischemia modified albumin (IMA) and albumin adjusted-IMA (AAIMA) as biomarkers for diabetic retinopathy. *Nepal J Ophthalmol.* 2015 Jul;7(14):117-23. doi: 10.3126/nepjoph.v7i2.14960. PubMed PMID: 27363956.
6. Seshadri Reddy V, Sethi S, Gupta N, Agrawal P, Chander Siwach R. Significance of Ischemia-Modified Albumin as a Simple Measure of Oxidative Stress and Its Discriminatory Ability in Diabetic Retinopathy: *Literature Review and Meta-Analysis. Retina.* 2016 Jun;36(6):1049-57. doi:10.1097/IAE.0000000000001042. Review. PubMed PMID: 27105326.

Chapter 4

COMPARISON OF IDEALISTIC COMMITMENTS BETWEEN FIRST AND THIRD YEAR MEDICAL STUDENTS

*Sabrina F. Merino, Lorena E. López Balbuena,
Ana María Rancich*, Ricardo J. Gelpi
and Martín Donato*
Institute of Cardiovascular Physiopathology
Department of Pathology, Faculty of Medicine,
University of Buenos Aires, Buenos Aires, Argentina

ABSTRACT

Introduction: Medicine is a career that could attract students with humanistic ideals. Idealism in medicine is understood as the pursuit of improved quality of life and relief of suffering for humankind, with emphasis on underserved populations. Several works have demonstrated that idealism decreases as the students' progress in their career, partially due to the hidden curriculum. The aim of this study is to compare first and

---

* Corresponding Author's E-mail: arancich@fmed.uba.ar.

third year medical students' commitments in relation to idealism and analyze their differences.

Material and methods: We administered an anonymous and voluntary survey to first and third year medical students of an Argentine university. The students had to answer demographic questions first and then write a maximum of 7 ethical compromises they would like to commit to as graduates. Only those commitments related to idealism were selected. The analysis between the variables was performed with the chi square test (P<0,05).

Results: A total of 1497 ethical commitments were obtained in first year and 1402 in third year. Out of those, 263 (17.6%) and 118 (8.4%) commitments, in first and third year respectively, were related to idealism. They referred to: the principle of justice and working with underserved populations; be a committed physician doing more than required; not use the medical profession as means for profit; follow ethics and morals and be an example for others; improve public health; be loyal to one's beliefs; obey the law and fight for human rights; save lives. The formulation of these commitments decrease in third year, being the relation between the variables was statistically significant ($X^2 = 27.47$; P $=0.0003$).

Discussion: Our results show a decrease in the formulation of idealistic commitments in third year that could be attributed to the hidden curriculum. Possible explanations could be the increased exposure to the medical profession, through the exchange of stories and anecdotes with professors and peers. Having taken the subject Bioethics and learning about Principialism with emphasis in patient's autonomy could have led third year students to express commitments more related to the doctor-patient relationship in particular and less with society in general. Also, the study of biomedical sciences and the lack of humanistic disciplines (only Bioethics and Mental Health during the first three years) would create a more technical mindset in the students, leaving aside issues related to the medical responsibility towards society.

Conclusion: Our study suggests that there is a decline in students' idealism in the first three years of medical school possibly due to the hidden curriculum.

Keywords: medical students, idealism, ethical commitments

INTRODUCTION

Medicine is a career in which not only biological but also humanistic contents converge, attracting students who, besides wishing an intellectual challenge, also possess humanitarian commitments. Idealism is understood as the belief that ideals are those principles that set high behavioral standards to be reached [1, 2]. There are authors who understand idealism as the perception of the world in a positive manner with the potential of achieving something good [3]. Particularly in medicine, it is usually related with seeking to improve the quality of life and alleviate the suffering of humanity, with an emphasis in providing medical attention focused on the service, care for underserved populations and concern for the health of society in general [4].

Upon entering the career, students feel the need to help the most vulnerable populations and a responsibility towards society. As years go by, however, they start to see the profession in a more cynical manner [5]. It has been attributed to the hidden curriculum, that which the institution teaches unconsciously and unintentionally, as one of the reasons for the decline of idealism [6, 7]. The hidden curriculum is a qualitative aspect of teaching, related with the transmission of knowledge, cognitive and psycho-motor abilities through attitudes, values and omissions, dependent on teachers but not explicit in official programs. The hidden curriculum can have a positive or negative influence on the students, and sometimes it can be contrary to the educational plans [8].

International articles have demonstrated that the desire of the students to assist underserved populations and be useful to society increases in those who participate in volunteering programs in poor areas of developing countries [9]. The University of Buenos Aires has students not only from Argentina but also from other countries of Latin America, currently mainly from Brazil. It is a fact that in many of these countries healthcare is concentrated in big cities, leaving large areas with precarious access to health [10, 11]. Being exposed to this reality in their countries of origin could contribute to many students starting a career with the goal of improving this situation.

In the first years of medicine in our university, the students take mainly biologicist subjects and they do not have contact with patients. The only humanistic subjects are Mental Health and Bioethics. In the latter, they learn the principles and rules of Principialism and the students are encouraged to think of the patient as an autonomous bio-psico-social-spiritual being. During these first three years, those students who have any sort of contact with patients, have it extracurricularly, by volunteering in Emergency Departments, working in healthcare or other volunteering activities. Literature demonstrates that when the student is exposed to clinical situations, idealism decreases in relation to the profession and patients, although they state that maybe what decreases is ingenuity [12].

It has been seen as well that those physicians with stronger religious convictions possess higher levels of idealism [3]. It has also been noted that there is a strong desire of the students to hold on to their personalities and elements of themselves (idealism, innocence, optimism), as they perceive that medical school tries to dehumanize them [13].

The literature that relates idealism with medical students comes mainly from Anglo-Saxon countries, being those articles from Latin America underrepresented. Therefore we thought it would be of interest to analyze and compare two populations of medical students in different moments of their career, determine if there is a decrease in idealism in pre-clinical years, and if there is any difference between those students from different Latin American nationalities. The aim of the present study is to analyze and compare the idealistic commitments of first and third year medical students of the University of Buenos Aires and between students of different Latin American nationalities. Another objective is to analyze if those commitments differ between the students in relation to age, gender, if they have contact with patients, if they are behind in their studies, if they work, and if they practice any religion.

MATERIAL AND METHODS

A voluntary and anonymous survey was administered to first and third year medical students of the University of Buenos Aires, Argentina. They were provided with a definition of what constitutes an ethical commitment: "The structure comprised by values, norms and healthy habits that justify human behavior in certain circumstances" [14]. They were asked to provide demographic information (age, gender, nationality, current year of medical school, if they work, if they have children, if they have relationship with patients, if they took the subject bioethics and in which year, if they profess any religion and they practice it, and year they entered medical school). Next, they were asked to write seven ethical commitments they would like to follow once they graduate as physicians.

The ethical commitments expressed by the students were categorized and transcribed in a database along with the demographical data. For this manuscript, only those commitments that were traditionally considered idealistic, in relation to help underserved populations, improve public health, have an impeccable moral conduct and be an example for others, not profit with the profession and contribute to society in an selfless manner, beyond the scopes of the profession and doing more than required, were considered. These commitments are related to service for underserved populations and responsibility towards society in general, responding to the definitions of idealism stated in the introduction. Those commitments related to empathy were not taken into consideration for considering that they refer to the interpersonal relationship between physician and patient and not with society as a whole.

Crossings were made between the variables to establish relationships between the demographic characteristics expressed in the objectives and the ethical commitments written by the students. The statistical analysis was performed with the non-parametric test Chi square ($P<0.05$).

This research has the approval of the Ethics Committee of a hospital associated to the Faculty of Medicine.

RESULTS

A total of 325 surveys were obtained in first year, with a mean age of 23.1 years (SD = 4.53). In third year, 277 students completed the survey, with a mean age of 24.5 years (SD = 3.83). Most of the students were female, with similar percentages in both years. Also, most students were Argentine, with a third part of Brazilians in first year (Table 1).

Table 1. Comparison of demographical data between first and third year

Demographical data of the students	First year (%)	Third year (%)
Female	67.7	69.0
Argentines	60.3	84.8
Brazilians	29.2	8.3
Other Latin Americans	8.6	6.1
Do not work	61.2	54.9
Do not have children	95.4	96.0
Do not have relationship with patients	79.1	66.8
Took Bioethics	14.5	97.5
Behind in their studies	52.0	75.8
Catholics	43.4	49.5
Do not practice their religion	47.3	53.4

Furthermore, more than half the students of both years did not work, did not have children, and did not have a relationship with patients. Half of first year and three thirds of third year students were behind in their studies. The most prevalent religion was Catholicism. Only 14.5% of first year students took Bioethics while most of third year students (97.5%) took it, since they need the subject approved to be able to continue in the future with clinical training (Table 1).

A total of 1497 ethical commitments were obtained in first year and 1402 in third-year. Those commitments related to idealism were 263 (17.6%) in first year and 118 (8.4%) in third-year. The relation between the formulations of idealistic commitments in comparison with non-idealistic commitments was statistically significant (Table 2).

These commitments were categorized in relation to idealistic principles: justice and working with underserved populations; be a committed physician and do more than required; not use the medical profession as means for profit; follow ethics and be an example for others; improve public health; be loyal to one's beliefs; obey the law and fight for rights; save lives. The rest of the commitments mentioned by the students were related to the individual doctor-patient relationship, respect for colleagues, commitments to oneself and to society.

Table 2. Idealistic vs non-idealistic commitments written by first and third year medical students

Commitments	First year students N (%)	Third year students N (%)	Total N (%)
Idealistic	263 (17.6)	118 (8.4)	381 (13.1)
Non-idealistic	1234 (82.4)	1284 (91.6)	2518 (86.9)
Total	1497 (100)	1402 (100)	2899 (100)

$X^2 = 53.12$ P = 0.0001.

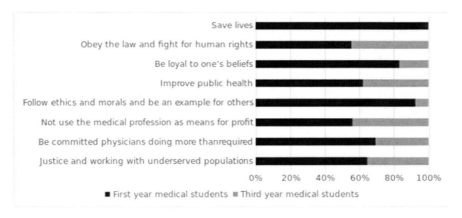

Figure 1. Idealistic commitments between first and third year medical students.

Also, when comparing only the idealistic commitments between students of different years, a decrease in third-year in the formulation of idealistic commitments is observed ("save lives" was absent). The relationship between both groups was statistically significant ($X^2 = 27.47$; P=0.0003) (Figure 1).

Furthermore, the students' idealistic commitments were related to other variables: age, gender, nationality, relationship with patients, being up-to-date or behind in their studies, professing or not professing a religion, practicing their religion or not in case of having one. None of these associations presented a significant relation in regards to the formulation of idealistic commitments. Conversely, when comparing the formulation of idealistic commitments of both groups together in relation to their country of origin, a statistical significance was found between Argentines, Brazilians and students from the rest of Latin America ($X^2 = 42.40$; P=0.0001). As it can be seen, "follow ethics and be an example for others" and "save lives" seem to be more prominent among Brazilian students (Figure 2).

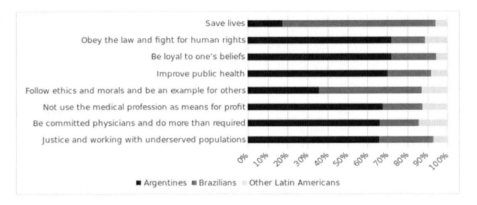

Figure 2. Idealistic commitments between medical students of different countries of origin.

DISCUSSION

Our results would reflect a decrease in the formulation of idealistic commitments in third year. This decrease, however, would not be related to other factors external to the university itself and the course of the career. Our findings are in concordance with some articles found in the literature, where it is demonstrated that there is a decrease in idealism throughout the career [15, 16]. Wolochuk et al. administered a questionnaire on attitudes toward social issues in medicine to students of different years. They demonstrated that as the students progressed in their studies, their attitudes toward social issues decreased. This decline was found at the end of pre-clinical studies (our equivalent to third year), with another decline at the end of the career.

These changes were attributed to the loss of the idealism that they possessed when initiating their studies and the hidden curriculum. In this same study, these attitudes are analyzed taking gender into consideration. They conclude that women are more idealistic than men [16]. Our results did not evidence a significant relation between the expression of idealistic commitments and the students' gender.

There are, however, differences between the results of this study in regards to others. In a work from Canada, the decrease of idealism in medical students is related with their exposure to a clinical setting and dealing with patients, disease and death, producing a change in the students' mentality, who leave aside medicine's humanistic principles to focus in objectivity and technology [17]. Conversely, our study would indicate that the decrease in idealism would be occurring before the systematic entry of the student in a clinical setting, since both first and third year medical students do not attend hospitals as part of the formal curriculum. Also, no significant relation was found among those students that had relationship with patients beyond school, whether for work or different types of volunteering activities with those that did not have contact with patients.

Another study analyzed through a survey, idealism in physicians from different cultures, taking into consideration their religious beliefs. They concluded that those with higher levels of religiosity were more idealistic [3]. Our results did not evidence significant relations between the beliefs and the religious practices of the students with the expression of idealistic commitments.

We speculated that there could have been a relation between idealism and the students' age, with a decrease in idealism as they gained more life experience, and became perhaps more realistic. However, we found no significant difference between these variables. It was also thought that those students who were behind in their studies would express less idealistic commitments since they already encountered difficulties with the study of the career and the profession, whether these were due to difficulty in comprehending concepts or for personal issues outside of school. However, we did not find either significant relations between these variables.

One of the possible reasons why there is significant relation between the nationality of the students and the expression of idealistic commitments could be due to the fact that our school gives international students the opportunity the access a quality high level education free of charge, which could predispose them to a more optimistic view of reality. However, those students that decide to leave their countries of origin to look for a better future or education could be naturally more idealistic than those that choose another alternative.

While idealism decreases during the first years of the career, some studies affirm that there is a resurgence when students are close to graduation, being the initial lay idealism replaced by a professional idealism, with a more realistic (but not necessarily pessimistic) view of the profession [15, 18]. The initial conception of the physician as an agent who "saves lives" is set aside to give priority to other issues, as in our study, or is replaced by "alleviating suffering," taking into consideration the limitations of medicine [15].

The decrease of idealistic commitments in third year and the fact that no demographic variable presented significant relation with the expression of those commitments, would indicate that the hidden curriculum is the most relevant factor to explain this phenomenon. The increasing immersion of the student in the healthcare system through their interaction with peers and professors, where anecdotes and stories are usually exchanged, could also be a factor of the hidden curriculum to be considered. The study of biomedical sciences, combined with the lack of humanistic disciplines (only Bioethics and Mental Health during the first years) could be guiding the students towards a more scientific and technical view of medicine, leaving aside those problems that affect society as a whole. This could have led third year students to express commitments more related with the physician-patient relationship in particular instead of with society in general. It would be interesting for a future study to take into consideration students from the last years of the career to analyze if the phenomenon of a more realistic resurgence of idealism also occurs in our school.

CONCLUSION

The decrease of medical students' idealism during the first years of the career could be a consequence of the hidden curriculum. It would be important to maintain a constant dialogue between students and teachers, raising awareness on those professional behaviors or situations in the healthcare system that could negatively influence the students, so the initial lay idealism turns into professional idealism instead of cynicism.

REFERENCES

[1] Cambridge Dictionary. (Last access 4th June 2019). *Definition of idealism*. Available at https://dictionary.cambridge.org.

[2] Cambridge Dictionary. (Last access 4th June 2019). *Definition of ideal*. Available at https://dictionary.cambridge.org.

[3] Malloy, D. C., Sevigny, P. R., Hadjistavropoulos, T., Bond, K., Fahey McCarthy, E., Murakami, M., Paholpak, S., Shalini, N., Liu, P. L., Peng, H. (2012). Religiosity and Ethical ideology of Physicians: A Cross-Cultural study. *Journal of Religion and Health*, 53(1):244-54.

[4] Mader, E. M., Roseamelia, C., Morley, C. P (2014). The temporal decline of idealism in two cohorts of medical students at one institution. *BMC Medical Education*, 14(58).

[5] Morley, C. P., Roseamelia, C., Smith, J. A., Villarreal, A. L. (2013). Decline of medical student idealism in the first and second year of medical school: a survey of pre-clinical medical students at one institution. *Medical Education Online*, 18 (21194).

[6] Stanek, A., Chantalle, C., Dylan Bould, M., Writer, H., Doja, A. (2015). Life imitating art: Depictions of the hidden curriculum in medical television programs. *BMC Medical Education*, 15(156).

[7] Wiecha, J. M., Markuns, J. F. (2008). Promoting Medical Humanism: Design and Evaluation of an Online Curriculum. *Family medicine*, 40(9):617-9.

[8] Rojas, A. (2012). "Currículum oculto" en medicina: una reflexión docente. *Revista Médica de Chile*, 140: 1213-1217. [Rojas, A. (2012). "Hidden curriculum" in medicine: a teacher's reflection. *Chilean Medical Journal*, 140:1213-1217].

[9] Smith, J. K., Weaver, D. B. (2006). Capturing medical students' idealism. *Annals of Family Medicine*, 4(Suppl 1): S32-S37.

[10] Departamento de Operación de evaluaciones del Banco Mundial. (1999). La atención de la salud en Brasil: el tratamiento de situaciones. *Précis*, Primavera 1999 (189):1-7. [Department of Operation evalations of the World Bank. (1999). Healthcare in Brazil: treatment of situations. *Précis*, spring 1999 (189): 1-7].

[11] Ministerio de Salud y Desarrollo Social. (Last access 9th June 2019). *Datos sobre fuerza de trabajo.* Available at: https://www.argentina.gob.ar/salud/oferhus/datos/fuerzadetrabajo.
[Ministry of Health and Social Development. (Last access 9th June 2019). *Data on the workforce.* Available at: https://www.argentina.gob.ar/salud/oferhus/datos/fuerzadetrabajo].

[12] Griffith, C. H., Wilson, J. F. (2001). The loss of student idealism in the 3rd-year clinical clerkships. *Evaluation & the Health Professions*, 24(1):61-71.

[13] Poirier, S., Ahrens, W. R., Brauner, D. J. (1998). Songs of innocence and experience: student's poems about their medical education. *Academic Medicine*, 73(5):473-8.

[14] Riera Ruza, L., Sansevero de Suarez, I. (2013). El compromiso ético del estudiante universitario en las experiencias de aprendizaje-servicio. *Omnia*: 19(11): 31-42. [Riera Ruza, L., Sansevero de Suarez, I. (2013). The ethical commitment of the university student in the experiences of learning-service. *Omnia*: 19(11): 31-42].

[15] Gutierrez-Medina, S., Cuenca-Gómez, D., Álvarez de Toledo, O. (2008). "Por qué quiero ser médico? *Educación Médica*. 11(1): S1-S6. [Gutierrez-Medina, S., Cuenca-Gómez, D., Álvarez de Toledo, O. (2008). Why do I want to be a physician? *Medical Education*, 11 (1): S1-S6].

[16] Woloschuk, W., Harasym, P. H., Temple, W. (2004). Attitude change during medical school: a cohort study. *Medical Education*, 38: 522–534.
[17] Neumann, M., Edelhäuser, F., Tauschel, D., Fischer, M. R., Wirtz, M., Woopen, C., Haramati, A., Scheffer, C. (2011). Empathy delcine and its reasons: a systematic review of studies with medical students and residents. *Academic Medicine*, 86(8): 996-1009.
[18] Becker, H. S., Geer, B. (1958). The fate of idealism in medical school. *American Sociological Review, 23(1):* 50-56.

BIOGRAPHICAL SKETCHES

Sabrina Fernanda Merino

Affiliation: Institute of Cardiovascular Physiopathology (INFICA), Department of Pathology, School of Medicine, University of Buenos Aires.

Education: Physician, School of Medicine, University of Buenos Aires

Business Address: J. E. Uriburu 950, 2nd Floor, Section A. C1114AAD Buenos Aires. Argentina

Lorena Elizabeth López Balbuena

Affiliation: Institute of Cardiovascular Physiopathology (INFICA), Department of Pathology, School of Medicine, University of Buenos Aires.

Education: Medical student, School of Medicine, University of Buenos Aires

Business Address: J.E Uriburu 950, 2nd Floor, Section A. C1114AAD Buenos Aires. Argentina

Ana María Rancich

Affiliation: Institute of Cardiovascular Physiopathology (INFICA), Department of Pathology, School of Medicine, University of Buenos Aires.

Education: Doctor in Medical Humanities, University of Buenos Aires.

Business Address: J.E Uriburu 950, 2nd Floor, Section A. C1114AAD Buenos Aires. Argentina

Research and Professional Experience: Human resources advisor, Institute of Cardiovascular Physiopathology (INFICA)

Ricardo J. Gelpi

Affiliation: Institute of Cardiovascular Physiopathology (INFICA), Department of Pathology, School of Medicine, University of Buenos Aires.

Education: Medical Doctor, School of Medicine, National University of La Plata.

Business Address: J.E Uriburu 950, 2nd Floor, Section A. C1114AAD Buenos Aires. Argentina

Research and Professional Experience:
   Dean, School of Medicine, University of Buenos Aires.
   Director, Pathology Department, School of Medicine, University of Buenos Aires.
   Director, Institute of Cardiovascular Physiopathology (INFICA), Department of Pathology, School of Medicine, University of Buenos Aires.
   Main Researcher, Scientific and Technical Research National Council (CONICET), Institute of Cardiovascular Physiopathology (INFICA)

Martín Donato

Affiliation: Institute of Cardiovascular Physiopathology (INFICA), Department of Pathology, School of Medicine, University of Buenos Aires.

Education: Medical Doctor, University of Buenos Aires.

Business Address: J.E Uriburu 950, 2nd Floor, Section A. C1114AAD Buenos Aires. Argentina

Research and Professional Experience: Pathology Associate Professor, Department of Pathology, School of Medicine, University of Buenos Aires. Associate research of the Scientific and Technical Research National Council (CONICET) and Institute of Cardiovascular Physiopathology (INFICA).

Chapter 5

CAN CODE SWITCHING COMPLEMENT LEARNING? SAUDI ARABIAN MEDICAL STUDENTS' PERCEPTIONS OF ENGLISH AS THE LANGUAGE OF INSTRUCTION

Mohammed Alenezi[1,*] *and Paul Kebble*[2]

[1]Ministry of Education, Kingdom of Saudi Arabia
[2]Coordinator of English Language Development,
Faculty of Health Sciences, Curtin University, Bentley WA, Australia

ABSTRACT

English language plays a crucial role in the delivery of medical education globally due to the vast body of medical related resources available only in English. This is clearly visible with most colleges and universities around the world offering medical and health science courses exclusively in English. Simultaneously textbooks and reference learning materials for medical education are available only in English. To benefit from this linguistic trend, Saudi Arabian education authorities have

---

[*] Corresponding Author's Email: Mohammed3062@hotmail.com.

incorporated English as the language of instruction for medical education in the Kingdom. To meet the learning and teaching requirements, along with Saudi Arabian academics teaching faculty in the Kingdom's medical colleges have been recruited from a variety of countries including USA, UK, South Africa, India, Egypt, Sudan, Syria and Pakistan. With English being the supposed sole medium of instruction within the classrooms, the linguistic expectations of these recruits is a proven high level of competency in English. The faculty members from Saudi Arabia and from other Arab countries, however, often prefer to mix English and Arabic in their linguistic medium of instruction and interaction in their teaching. From a learner's perspective, it requires noting that English, being a foreign language in the Kingdom of Saudi Arabia, poses diverse challenges to Saudi medical students. As a language of instruction and interaction inside the classroom, the switching between English and Arabic receives mixed reactions from both instructors and students. The engaged code-switching (English-Arabic/ Arabic-English) is perceived to be beneficial by some, while others view it as a substantial obstacle in mastering the target language, English. This blended, interwoven linguistic relationship between English and Arabic inside some Saudi Arabian medical classrooms, along with the perceptions of teachers and students towards the same, are explored in the current paper. Using questionnaires as data collection instruments, the paper reports on the qualitative analysis of responses and subsequent discussion. This includes direct implications and consequential recommendations for Saudi Arabian medical education authorities to better achieve the objectives of medical education through the medium of English language instruction in the Kingdom of Saudi Arabia.

Keywords: medical students, Saudi learners, code-switching, medium of instruction, English as a foreign language

INTRODUCTION

Using English as the medium of instruction in higher education medical institutions across the Kingdom of Saudi Arabia has often been a topic of debate and research within the Kingdom. It should be initially noted that the teaching of the English Language in Saudi Arabia has its own history. According to Al-Seghayer (2011), the learning of English was introduced into the Kingdom's curriculum in 1928 with the aim of furnishing students with one of the world's living languages, and what Al-Hajailan (2003) describes as a tool to acquire knowledge with which to serve humanity. As Alrashidi and Phan (2015) report, English has now become a compulsory medium of instruction in most universities within the Kingdom. Presently, Saudi educational policymakers have mandated English as the Medium of Instruction in all higher education institutions across the kingdom. However, Arabic, being the mother tongue of Saudi students, is the only medium of instruction in schools up to secondary level, although English is taught as a foreign language from 4th grade elementary school (Alrashidi and Phan, 2015). It is only at the undergraduate level that English officially gets introduced as the language of instruction. This language shift in instruction can become an obstacle to effective learning, creating issues of confusion and subsequent disengagement with, and rejection of, the new linguistic medium of instruction. From the perspectives of Saudi Higher Education (HE) policy makers, there has been a significant educational trends towards providing most courses through the medium of English. This is seen as facilitating the accelerated and broadening use of English to create what Graddol (1997) refers to as a constituency of HE graduates who will continue to use English extensively amongst themselves. Witnessing the worldwide acceptance of English as an international language and its implementation as a medium of instruction, Saudi Arabia has also approved an honoured status to English language instruction in educational institutions across the country. For example, Al-Jarf (2008) reports that in the colleges of medicine, pharmacy, science, and computer science of the acclaimed King Saud University, English is the endorsed language of learning and teaching.

The concept of employing English as the medium of instruction is supported by scholars such as Coleman (2006) and Zare-ee & Gholami (2013) who argue that it develops learners' proficiency in English, subsequently enhancing career opportunities through improved mobility, along with further study abroad opportunities. Belhiah and Elhami (2015) through their research focused on teachers and learners from six universities in the United Arab Emirates, reported that teachers and learners were overall positive towards the use of English as a Medium of Instruction. However, it is essential to note that while teachers and students described the positives of English as a Medium of Instruction, its efficacy in enhancing students' English language proficiency is unclear. Moreover, the obligatory implementation of English as a medium of instruction without considering; a) learners' and teachers' language proficiency, b) the dearth of resources, c) suitable support systems, and d) a lack of competent teachers to conduct English as a Medium of Instruction classes, have resulted in numerous challenges and adverse consequences for student learning and engagement.

On the other hand, contemporary research has revealed strong arguments for the use of first language in supporting instruction and learning in a second language. The notion has fostered recommendations of its controlled use in what Machaal (2012) refers to as a cognitive and mediating tool in teaching and learning in the target language. Swain and Lapkin (2000) recognise the use of L1 as an important cognitive tool in carrying out tasks that are cognitively and linguistically complex. In addition, Eldridge (1996) argues that there is no first-hand confirmation to support the idea that restricting mother tongue use would essentially improve learning efficiency. He argues that using both languages, code-switching, in the target language classroom can be highly purposeful and relevant to pedagogical goals.

With a focus on HE lecturers engaged in teaching in the Kingdom of Saudi Arabia, it can be seen that the educational system in the Kingdom of Saudi Arabia, particularly at the university level, reveals the predominance of three categories of lecturers: 1) English speaking teachers with English as a first language, 2) Arab teachers with English as an additional language, and 3) teachers from Asian countries such as India and Pakistan with English as one of multiple first languages or as an additional language (Khan, 2011). Khan (2011) argues that native English teachers cannot use bilingual strategies to teach, the native Arab teachers are ineffective because of their traditional Grammar Translation Method of learning and teaching, with the third group of teachers not aware of the realities of the Saudi Arabian context.

These described complexities in the use of English as a medium of instruction within the Saudi Arabian medical student context, along with consideration of the direct views and attitudes of the teachers and learners engaged with using English as their medium of instruction within the classrooms, are explored further within this chapter.

LITERATURE REVIEW

Language Policy in the Kingdom of Saudi Arabia

Language policy plays a decisive role in the designing of effective education policies. In the Kingdom of Saudi Arabia, Arabic, being the official and native language, is the principal spoken language, and is greatly influenced by religion. The Kingdom is therefore virtually a monolingual country, outside of education. As Arabic is the language of the Holy Quran, the Saudi government intends to preserve the sanctity of the religion, heritage, and culture directly through the Arabic language. The Saudi education policy provides five articles (24, 46, 50, 114, 140) related to language policy (Al-Abdaly, 2012). These articles stipulate that all educational levels should be taught in Arabic to enrich the Arabic language by improving the linguistic ability of all its citizens and a resultant focus on Arabization. There are also provisions, in articles 50, to acquire knowledge from another language in order to promote Arabization, spread knowledge among the citizens, contribute to Islam, and to serve humanity. To achieve the acquisition of knowledge in other languages, the Saudi Ministry of Education passed a law in 2003 mandating the teaching of English in public schools starting from Grade six. And a year later, the teaching of English started in Grade five (Al-Jarf, 2008) and subsequently in Grade 4 (Alrashidi and Phan, 2015).

Focusing on students' perspectives on the medium of instruction, Al-Seghayer (2012) reported that some students preferred Arabic over English as a medium of instruction while other did not see any real difference in either of the two. Some students suggested that having more text books translated into Arabic we be more conducive to effective teaching in Arabic. According to Al-Seghayer (2012), article 50 of the Saudi Educational Policy stipulates that students should learn at least one foreign language, this being the rationale for English teaching in Saudi schools, where the learners' ability to communicate with international language users ranks as a priority. In practical terms, numerous private and international schools with English as their medium of education are thriving across the kingdom. Originally to cater for the educational needs of the children of the expatriate workers in the kingdom, the private institutions are increasingly attracting Saudi students wishing to have greater exposure to English.

However, even though the Saudi government is investing billions of Dollars in the promotion of learning in English language medium, or the learning of English, the language still has a very restricted use in Saudi society. The English language has a very limited purpose in the everyday lives of Saudis as they invariably use the Arabic language at home as well as in their interactions with friends, peers, and work colleagues.

Code-Switching, Code-Blending and L1 Usage

The term 'Code' implies language varieties, styles and mixed languages. Romaine (1995) believes that code is confined not only to different languages but also to varieties of languages and styles. However, Myers-Scotton (2006) considers code as a cover term for separate languages, dialects and styles. In addition to this, Rahman and Hossain (2012) add some categories of mixed languages to the range of code. According to Appel and Muysken (2005, p. 117), it is that manifestation of bilingual interaction where the lexical and grammatical properties of one language are incorporated into the 'utterances' of another language. In the words of Poplack and Meechan (1998), code mixing is 'any use of two or more languages in the same discourse' (p. 127).

In learning and teaching utilising the medium of a language additional to the learners' mother tongue, the engagement of the most proficient common language is inevitable. This can occur in three key ways, through code-switching, code-blending and the use of learners' L1 to augment understanding.

Code-Switching describes when communicators fluctuate between sentences provided in multiple languages, often two. In the author's experience, sitting in a restaurant in Malaysia it is common to hear a conversation move between English, Malay and Hokkien (or other Chinese dialect). Those engaged in the conversation will understand that certain nuances are best described in given languages. Simply put, if the conversation is focused on Chinese food, the language used will predominantly be a Chinese dialect, if world politics is being discussed, this could well be in English, and if local politics are addressed, then Malay could well be engaged. This can equally be demonstrated in the classroom where concepts that have been introduced in the medium of English will often be discussed in English, however, subsequent notions that have a local bias may well be discussed in the L1. Again, in the author's professional experience lecturing in the UAE, broader conversations and discussions were invariably conducted in English, with more personal break-out discussions often reverting to Arabic. Code-blending happens when specific lexical items are referred to in L1 even though the conversation is being conducted in L2. This may be due to either the speaker not knowing the L2 translation of the item or just for convenience. Conversely, L1 may be being used with L2 vocabulary interspliced. Code-blending, therefore, happens at word level and not sentence level.

Students who are learning in L2 may have a specific comprehension issue that an instantaneous translation in L1 would alleviate. A student colleague, or maybe the lecturer, may well be in a position to provide the translation or explanation as a shortcut to understanding. In this author's experience, this notion is contentious in terms of being a supported practise in learning and teaching, although the personal experiential understanding is that its limited use can be advantageous. In this chapter the phrase 'code-mixing' will be used as an inclusive term for all of the above concepts.

Code-Switching in the Medical Classrooms: Related Studies

In international medical education, using a foreign language for instruction can pose many difficulties, that is why the Syrian government, for example, has opted to use Arabic as the medium of Instruction in their Medical schools (GHOBAIN, 2015). However, according to Alshareef, Osama, Mohamud, Alrajhi, Alhamdan and Hamad. (2018), most Medical Schools in Arab-speaking countries have selected English as the medium of instruction. Studies within Arab countries have reported that there are both communication and cultural gaps between students and instructors in a typical lecture delivered in English. These factors often result in code-mixing to mitigate the frictions of the foreign language as the medium of instruction, with Arabic being engaged in, often for topic-related explanations, leading to clearer comprehension.

Focusing on the research on the feasibility of using Arabic as a medium of instruction at colleges of medicine, Al-Jarallah and Al-Ansari (1998) reported that 60% of medical students at King Saud University in Saudi Arabia preferred Arabic as a medium of instruction. In another study conducted by Al-Mohandes and Baker (1998) across all faculties, 66% of the students at King Saud University favoured the use of both Arabic and English in delivering class lectures. 57% of the students preferred to use Arabic textbooks, 53% preferred to write their projects in Arabic, while 39% preferred to answer test questions in Arabic. On the other hand, in the Faculty of Engineering, only 22% preferred to use English in delivering class lectures, 32% preferred to use English engineering textbooks, 33% preferred to write their engineering projects in English, and 44% preferred to answer test questions in English.

In an earlier study, Assuhaimi and Al-Barr (1992) reported that 77% of medical students at King Faisal University in Saudi Arabia favoured answering test questions in Arabic as opposed to 23% who wished to answer test questions in English. In Al-Jarallah and Al-Ansari's (1998) study, almost 90% of the students informed that they comprehended more when lectures were delivered in both English and Arabic through the mixture of codes. Al-Sebaee (1995) researched two experimental groups of Arab medical students at the American University of Beirut and Jordan University in Amman. The results revealed that the medical students saved 50% of their time through reading medical textbooks in Arabic.

A later study by Al-Jarf (2004) investigated college students' attitudes towards using English and Arabic as a medium of instruction at the university level. The findings indicated that most participants considered English more appropriate for teaching medicine, pharmacy, engineering, science, nursing, and computer science. In a similar study by Alenezi (2010) investigating students' language attitudes towards Arabic and English code-switching as the medium of instruction of a science subject in Kuwait University, it was revealed that students had a strong preference toward a specific medium of instruction utilising Arabic/English code switching. The results clearly showed students' positive language attitudes towards the engagement of code switching in learning and teaching. A study by Alenezi and Kebble (2018) investigated attitudes of Saudi medical students' todawrds English-Arabic code-switching in classroom activities. The results revealed that students described their 'increased repect for the lecturers practising code-switching' (p.143). With such conflicting views and attitudes of students about the use of English as a Medium of Instruction, this study attempted to explore the perceptions of Saudi Arabian medical students.

METHODOLOGY

The study employed quantitative approach using students-questionnaire as data collection instrument. The data collected were analysed using SPSS to determine the quantitative results gained from the questionnaire. This methodology was instigated on the basis of being able to substantiate any potential changes to institutional pedagogy as Creswell (2008) argues results from a quantitative research methodology have the potential to be generalised to larger populations.

Participates

The participants of this study were medical students of the Northern Border University in Saudi Arabia. The total number of the students who participated in the study was 230 students, 127 male and 103 female, whose ages ranged from 18 to 23.

Data Collection Instrument

For quantitative analysis, the main data collection instrument was the questionnaire (see Appendix A). Questionnaires are an inexpensive way to gather data from a potentially large number of respondents. Cohen, Manion, Morrison & Morrison (2007) explain further that the questionnaire is a very useful instrument for the collection of information, and can be administered in the absence of the researcher.

In the present study, the questionnaire was adopted from the Alenezi (2010) investigation into students' attitudes towards code switching. The questionnaire (appendix 1) is divided into two major sections. The first section of the questionnaire requires demographical information from the students such as gender, language taught in previous school and language use as a medium of instruction in the class. Section two of the questionnaire contains 13 items asking for specific information in relation to the linguistic medium of learning and teaching. The first 4 items of the questionnaire focused on the students' attitude toward code-switching. The items 5, 6 and 7 focus on participants' knowledge of their first and second languages. The items 8, 9 and 10 focus on participants' opinion of their instructors based on the use of languages in teaching. The last 3 items (11, 12 and 13) focus on participants' opinion of their academic results based on the languages used in the class room.

Data Collection Procedures

Adhering to research ethics, necessary verbal approval from the instructors of the medical faculty of Northern Border University in Arar, Saudi Arabia was obtained prior to distributing questionnaires to students. Verbal approval from each participant was also obtained. The questionnaire was administered to the students after a brief introductory talk in which the procedure was clearly explained. Moreover, the participants were encouraged to ask questions at any time during the administration of the questionnaire. The students took between 15 and 20 minutes to complete the questionnaire. The participants' particulars were kept confidential and it was optional for their names to be written on the questionnaire.

Data Analysis

For analysing the data collected from participants through the questionnaires, the Statistical Package for Social Sciences (SPSS) version 16 was used. Descriptive statistics were employed to explore, summarise and describe the data. Pallant (2007) states that descriptive statistic is aimed at depicting the different attributes of data, verifying any violation of the principal assumptions for the statistical methods to be used in the study, and addressing particular research questions. In this study, the descriptive statistics were undertaken using central tendency and variation statistics including frequency, means, ranges, and standard deviation.

Pilot Study

According to Zikmund (2003), a pilot test is an experimental study aimed at enhancing particular research instrumentations. Thus, it was deemed useful for this study to conduct a pilot test in order to increase the accuracy and consistency of the measurements. According to Hunt, Sparkman, and Wilcox (1982), the sample size for a pilot test is at least 30.

In response, this study managed to randomly employ a sample of 35 students from Northern Border University. The returned responses were 33 questionnaires, with two exempted from the analysis through too many questions left unanswered, with a final 31 questionnaires used for analytical purposes. The pilot study was employed to test face and construct validity as well as conduct initial reliability analysis. Each is discussed in the following sections and with reference to Table 1.

Table 1. Cronbach Alpha Analysis

Variable	No items	Cronbach Alpha
Attitude	1-2-3-4	0.798
L1 and L2	5-6-7	0.871
Teachers image	8-9-10	0.801
Results	11-12-13	0.750
Code switching	5 to 13	0.819

Validity and Reliability

Adcock & David (2001) in Sekaran & Bougie (2010) cited that construct validity refers to the degree in which the construct measured is unbiased and ensured consistent measurement across time and across various items in the instrument. The reliability of measure is a sign of stability and consistency in which the instrument measures the concept and assesses the integrity of the measurement (Sekaran, & Bougie, 2010, p.162).

Face validity is the degree to which a test appears to measure what it claims to measure. Pilot testing revealed that the questions did not cause problems for students in terms of language and clarity.

The study was conducted using the Likert-Scale questionnaire. When the items on an instrument are not scored 'right' versus 'wrong', Cronbach's alpha is often used to measure the internal consistency. Cronbach alpha is an index of reliability for quantitative data that is generally used by researchers to ascertain how well the items in a set are positively correlated. The closer the value of cronbach alpha to one, the higher the internal consistency reliability. In general, reliabilities less than 0.60 are considered to be poor, those are in 0.70 ranges acceptable, and over 0.80 good (Sekaran & Bougie, 2010, p.325).

The reliability of measure is a sign of stability and consistency in which the instrument measures the concept and assesses the goodness of measure (Sekaran & Bougie, 2010). Theoretically, initial internal consistency reliability is assessed on the pilot data using Cronbach's alpha (Cronbach, 1984). Then, a more detailed reliability analysis is performed on the complete data set, in which a high reliability coefficient indicates a highly reliable instrument. Nunnally (1978) recommends that Cronbach's alpha value must be greater than 0.7 to show high reliability. The results revealed that all items for Attitude (alpha = 0.798) and Code Switching (alpha = 0.819) are included because they meet the conditions. As a summary, all reliability is exhibited in Table 2.

Table 2. Scale reliability alpha – pilot test

Variable	Factor	No Items	Cronbach's Alpha	Overall Cronbach's Alpha
Attitude	Attitude	4	0.798	0.798
Code Switching	First language and second language	3	0.781	0.819
	Teachers Images	3	0.801	
	Results	3	0.756	

FINDINGS

The study employed an initial sample of 230 students from Northern Border University of whom 194 returned completed questionnaires. Five of these questionnaires were excluded from the analysis as they contained too many unanswered questions. Therefore a total of 189 questionnaires were finally analysed and, from the responses, the following recapitulation frequency table was constructed (Table 3), and presented as a table of percentages.

Table 3. Saudi Medical Students' Attitudes towards Code-Switching

No	Statement	SD (%)	DA (%)	A (%)	SA (%)	M	Ratio % Dis - Ad
Attitude of Students							
1	Teaching the course only in one language is beneficial to me.	9.5	12.2	49.2	29.1	2.9788	21.7 - 78.3
2	Teaching the course in Arabic and English is desirable to me.	0	0	69.8	30.2	3.3016	0 - 100
3	Teaching the course in Arabic and English makes it easy for me to understand.	0	0	69.3	30.7	3.3069	0 - 100
4	It confuses me when course instructor teaches in Arabic and English in the same class period.	22.2	70.4	7.4	0	1.8519	92.6 - 7.4
Attitudes towards Instructors based on the use of languages in teaching							
5	I respect an instructor more when teaching in Arabic and English.	0	0	50.8	49.2	3.4921	0 - 100
6	I respect an instructor more when teaching in Arabic.	7.4	9.6	46	37	3.1270	17 - 83
7	I respect an instructor more when teaching in English.	7.4	7.9	45.5	39.2	3.1640	15.3 - 84.7
Attitudes based on academic results based on language used in the classroom							
8	Teaching the course only in Arabic increases my chances of passing the exams.	0	18	43.4	38.6	3.2063	18 - 82
9	Teaching the course only in English increases my chances of passing the exams.	2.6	14.3	41.8	41.3	3.2169	16.9 - 83.1
10	Teaching the course in Arabic and English increases my chances of passing the exams.	0	9	43.9	47.1	3.3810	9 - 91

Note: SD (strongly disagree); DA (disagree); A (agree); SA (strongly agree); M (mean).

Medical Students' Attitudes towards Code-Switching

Teaching the Course Only in One Language Is Beneficial to Me
   The majority of students agreed with teaching using one language. A total of 78.3% students (148) agreed or strongly agreed, with 21.7% (51) students strongly disagreeing. Although the language of instruction was not specified, this result suggests students appreciate the linguistic consistency that learning and teaching in one language can offer.

Teaching the Course in Arabic and English Is Desirable to Me
   69.8% (132) of the students agreed and 30.2% (57) students strongly agreed, i.e., all students were positive that they learned more when teaching was provided in both Arabic and English.

Teaching the Course in Arabic and English Makes It Easy for Me to Understand
   In support of further interpretations of the previous statement, belief that understanding was clearer when Arabic and English were combined as the linguistic medium of learning was measured. 69.3% (131) students agreed and 30.7 (58) students strongly agreed.

It Confuses Me When Course Instructor Teaches in Arabic and English in the Same Class Period
   The vast majority of students disagreed that confusion was caused by the use of English and Arabic in the same class period, with 92.6% (175) disagreeing and only 7.4% (14) students agreeing with the statement.

Medical Students' Attitudes towards Instructors Based on the Use of Languages in Teaching

I Respect Instructor More When Teaching in Arabic and English

50.8% (96) students agreed and 49.2% (93) students strongly agreed that their respect for the instructor will increase when the instructor is able to effectively utilise both Arabic and English in their learning and teaching.

I Respect Instructor More When Teaching in Arabic

83% (157) of the students agreed and 16.9% (32) students disagreed that they have more respect to the instructor when teaching in Arabic. It is likely that most of the students agreed with this because the students' first language is Arabic. Using Arabic will avoid confusion in teaching for all students especially for those who have inadequate mastery in English.

I Respect Instructor More When Teaching in English

84.7% (160) students agreed and 15.3% (29) students disagreed that their respect for the instructor will increase when the instructor teaches using English. In the authors' belief, this finding is not surprising because most English language learners understand the importance of being able to function within medicine in English. The majority of the students agreed with this item potentially because in using English, the students will learn more subject-specific English terminology.

Attitudes Based on Academic Results Based on Language Used in the Classroom

Teaching the Course in Arabic Increases My Chances of Passing the Exams

52.4% (99) of the students agreed and 47.6% (90) students strongly agreed that teaching the course in Arabic will increase the chances of passing the exam. It is potentially because teaching in Arabic or the students' first language will help the students to understand better and improve their grades.

Teaching the Course in English Increases My Chances of Passing the Exams

The vast majority of students, 83.1% (157), agreed that teaching the course in English will increase their chances of passing the exams, while 16.9% (32) students disagreed. As much medical terminology is in English, and the profession internationally relies on a high level of English competency, the exams incorporate much English. Students are well aware that English competency, therefore, will enhance their ability to be successful in these examinations.

Teaching the Course in Arabic and English Increases My Chances of Passing the Exams

80% (182) students agreed and 9% (17) students disagreed that by teaching the course in Arabic and English will increase their chances of passing the exams. A possible interpretation for this is that most of the students agreed that code-switching between English and Arabic will help them in improving their skills both in the first and second languages.

DISCUSSION

This study aimed to explore Arabic-speaking Saudi medical students' attitudes towards the use of code-switching between Arabic and English in learning and teaching. Overall, the results of the questionnaire showed positive attitudes towards the use of code-switching. These findings are consistent with Cook (2001); Alenezi (2010); Alenezi, (2016). Comparing the students' attitudes towards using one language (either Arabic or English) in teaching through Arabic-English code-switching, the findings of this study indicated the preference for using code-switching rather than using one language as a medium of instruction. Although the majority of the students strongly agreed that using one language is still beneficial to them, they found it more desirable and believed it makes the course material more easily understood if code-switching is utilised.

CONCLUSION

The study aimed to investigate Saudi medical students' attitudes towards code-switching for instruction purposes inside classrooms. The students' attitudes towards code-switching as a medium of instruction were very positive. They regard the use of both English and Arabic in learning and teaching as having a positive impact on their academic performance. It was regarded as an influential teaching tool to facilitate learning and to increase student comprehension resulting in their academic success. In summary, Saudi medical students at the Northern Border University, Saudi Arabia had positive attitudes towards the practice of code-switching between Arabic and English for instruction purposes. The students also demonstrated greater respect for the lecturers who practised code-switching during the class. This can be put further into context by considering that English is taught as a foreign language in Saudi Arabia and it is not easy for many students to comprehend difficult concepts in medical science purely in English without any supporting explanation in their mother tongue, Arabic. The study presents certain implications. Teachers will be better informed about the rationality of the judicious use of Arabic. Harmony between teachers and students is suggested so that teachers use Arabic for the required purposes, and not for every purpose. Thoughtful bilingual approach may boost the motivational level of Saudi Medical, specifically students with low proficiency level in English. Therefore, it is recommended that educational decision makers and managers at programs, department, colleges, and university levels in Saudi Arabia should consider revising their language policy in order to incorporate code-switching in the planning of syllabi.

REFERENCES

Al-Abdaly, A. H. *The Impact of English as a Medium of Instruction on Science Learning: Perception of the Medicine Female Students and Academic Staff at King Khalid University- A Thesis Submitted in Partial Fulfillment of the Requirements for the Master's Degree in Applied Linguistics.* Riyadh, Saudi Arabia. 2012.

Alenezi, A. "Students' language attitude towards using code-switching as a medium of instruction in the college of health sciences: An exploratory study." *ARECLS7*, 2010: 1–22.

Alenezi, M. "Gender and students' attitude toward code-switching: A correlational study with reference to Saudi Arabian medical students at Northern Border University." *International Journal of English Language & Translation Studies*.4 (3), 2016: 154–166.

Alenezi, M. and Kebble, P. "Investigating Saudi Medical Students' Attitudes towards English-Arabic Code-Switching in Classroom Instruction" *The Asian ESP Journal.* 14(1), 2018: 142-161.

Al-Hajailan, T. A. *Teaching English in Saudi Arabia.* Riyadh: Aldar Alsawlatia, 2003.

Al-Jarallah, H. & Al-Ansari, L. "Medical Students' Views of and Attitudes towards Teaching Medicine in Arabic." *Proceedings of the Arabization and Translation Development in Saudi Arabia. King Saud University.* Riyadh, 1998. 453-437.

Al-Jarf, R. "The Impact of English as an International Language (EIL) upon Arabic in Saudi Arabia." *The Asian EFL Journal, 10(4).* 2008:193-210.

Al-Muhandes, A. & Al-Hajj B. "Translation at King Saud University." *Proceedings of the Arabization and Translation Development in Saudi Arabia.* King Saud University, Riyadh. 1988.

Alrashidi, O. & Phan, H. "Education context and English teaching and learning in the Kingdom of Saudi Arabia: An Overview." *English Language Teaching, 8*(5). 2015: 33-44.

Al-Sebaee, Z. *Experiments in Using Arabic as a Medium of Instruction in Medical Schools.* Eastern Province Literary Association. Dammam, Saudi Arabia. 1995.

Al-Seghayer, K. *English Teaching in Saudi Arabia: Status, Issues, and Challenges*. Riyadh: Hala Print Co. 2011.

Al-Seghayer, K. *Status and functions of English in Saudi Arabia*. http://www.saudigazette.com.sa.11December2012. http://www.saudigazette.com.sa/index.cfm?method=home.regcon&contentid=20121211145659 (accessed May 05, 2019).

Alshareef, Musab, Osama Mobaireek, Mohamud Mohamud, Ziyad Alrajhi, Ali Alhamdan, and Bashir Hamad. *Decision Makers' Perspectives on the Language of Instruction in Medicine in Saudi Arabia: A Qualitative Study*. Health Professions Education 4, no. 4 (2018): 308-316.

Appel, R. & Muyesken, P. *Language Contact and Bilingualism*. London: Amsterdam University Press. 2005.

Assuhaimi, S. & Al-Barr, A. "Medical Students' Attitudes towards Medical Education." *Arabian Gulf Journal.* 1992.

Belhiah, H. & Elhami, M. "English as a Medium of Instruction in the Gulf: When Students and Teachers Speak." *Language Policy. 14.* 2015: 3-23.

Cohen, L., Manion, L., Morrison, K., & Morrison, K. R. B. *Research methods in education* (6th ed.). Psychology Press. 2007.

Coleman, J. A. "English Medium Teaching in European Higher Education." *Language Teaching.* 1. 2006: 1-14.

Cook, V. *Second Language Learning and Language Teaching* (3rd ed.). London: Arnold. 2001.

Creswell, J. *Educational Research: Planning, Conducting and Evaluating Quantitative and Qualitative Research* (3rd ed.). Lincoln University of Nebraska, Nebraska: Pearson Prentice Hall. 2008.

Ghobain, E. "Translation as a Scaffolding Teaching Strategy in English-medium Classrooms." *International Journal of Translation* Vol. 27, No. 1-2. 2015:1-16.

Graddol, D. The Future of English. In *A guide to forecasting the popularity of the English language in the 21st century.* London, UK: The British Council. 1997.

Khan, I. A. "The Teacher of English: Pedagogic Relevance in Saudi Arabia." *English Language Teaching, 4*(2). 2011: 112-120.

Machaal, B. "The use of Arabic in English Classes: A Teaching Support or a Learning Hindrance?" *Arab World English Journal, 3*(2). 2012. 194-231.

Myers-Scotton, C. *An Introduction to Bilingualism.* United Kingdom: Blackwell. 2006.

Northern Border University. *Northern Border University Handbook.* Arar: Northern Border University Press. 2009.

Pallant, J. *SPSS Survival Manual. (3rd ed.)* Philadelphia, PA: Open Press University, McGraw-Hill. 2007.

Poplack, S. & Meechan, M. Introduction: How Languages Fit together in Code- Mixing. *International Journal of Bilingualism, 2*(2). 1998: 127-138.

Rahman, S. & Hossain, R. "Code-Switching and Bilingualism: A Sociopsychological Study. *Journal of the Institute of Modern Languages, 23.* 2012: 233-248.

Sekaran, U. *& Bougie,* R. *Research Methods. For Business: A Skill Building Approach* (5th ed.). West. Sussex, UK: John Wiley & Sons Ltd. *2010.*

Swain, M., & Lapkin, S. "Task-Based Second Language Learning: The Use of the First Language." *Language Teaching Research, 4*(3). 2000: 251-174.

Zare-ee, A. & Gholami, K. "Academic Justifications for Preferring English as a Medium of Instruction by Iranian University Teachers." *Proceeding of the Global Summit on Education (GSE2013).* 2013: 11-12.

APPENDIX A: QUESTIONNAIRE

Introduction

This questionnaire is designed to find out your honest views about the language of teaching at your current course. Please respond to all the questions below carefully and honestly. This is not a test and there are no right or wrong answers. Your responses will be kept strictly confidential, and will only be used for the purpose of this study. Your answers will not prejudice you in any way.

Section A: Biographical Information

Please, answer the following questions.

1. What is your gender?
a. Female.
b. Male.

2. In what language(s) have you been mostly taught in your previous schooling?
a. Arabic.
b. English.
c. English and Arabic.

3. What language(s) do you use in communicating with your classmates, teachers, and staff at the college?
……………………………………………………………………..
……………………………………………………………………..
……………………………………………………………………..

Section B: Learners Honest Views About the Teaching Language

Please read each of the following statements very carefully and tick the answer which best describes your degree of agreement or disagreement. The following abbreviations are used: SA - Strongly Agree; AG - Agree; DA Disagree; SD - Strongly Disagree.

No	Item Description	SD (1)	DA (2)	AG (3)	SA (4)
1	Teaching the course only in one language is beneficial to me.				
2	Teaching the course in Arabic and English is desirable to me.				
3	Teaching the course in Arabic and English makes it easy for me to understand.				
4	It confuses me when course instructor teaches in Arabic and English at the same class period.				
5	I respect instructor more when teaching in Arabic and English.				
6	I respect instructor more when teaching in Arabic.				
7	I respect instructor more when teaching in English.				
8	Teaching the course in Arabic increases my chances of passing the exams.				
9	Teaching the course in English increases my chances of passing the exams.				
10	Teaching the course in Arabic and English increases my chances of passing the exams.				

In: Exploring the Opportunities ... ISBN: 978-1-53616-213-4
Editor: Elias A. Jespersen © 2019 Nova Science Publishers, Inc.

Chapter 6

SOCIAL SKILLS OF PHYSICIANS AND MEDICAL STUDENTS: PROBLEM OVERVIEW (FROM EXPERIENCE OF UKRAINE)

Lesya V. Lymar[*]
*Department of Foreign Languages,
National Medical University named after O. Bogomolets,
Kyiv, Ukraine*

ABSTRACT

The chapter describes the notion of the physician's social skills and their structure, with emphasis on shaping social skills in medical students during their medical studies. The paper deals with the peculiarities of medical social skills in Ukraine as a country the Health Service of which has undergone rather difficult changes after 1991. Social skills of a physician represent his knowledge, abilities and skills of productive interpersonal interaction with the patient, according to the standards accepted in the society and medical environment, which benefit both sides; good social skills are essential for a well-performing physician. It is a rare

---
[*] Corresponding Author's E-mail: lesyalymar@ukr.net.

case when the person enters Medical School with the already well-shaped social skills; social skills of a medical student usually need correction, in Ukraine particularly.

The following components within the structure of the physician's social skills have been defined: motivation, cognition, emotions, management and communication. Predominance of professional motives, combined with scientific and social motives, compose the efficient social skills' motivation component. The cognition component of social skills of the physician is represented with the physician's knowledge on the essence, factors and strategies of productive interaction with others. The management component of the physician's social skills is represented with various behavior practical abilities and skills of productive interaction, well-developed skills of self-analysis, etc. The emotional component of social skills, represented with the average "moderate" empathy expression, will provide for t productive interaction and prevention of conflicts. The communication component of social skills is represented with the physician's tendency to perceive the patient as an equal communication partner. All these components should be closely monitored in medical students and corrected throughout their medical studies, before they start their practice with the patients, using the methods described in the chapter.

Keywords: social skills, physician, doctor-patient interaction, medical students, medical schools

INTRODUCTION

The basic tasks of Medical School include providing medical students with the knowledge, abilities and skills required for performing their professional duties, which refers not only to teaching them at theoretical and practical classes, but shaping their professional abilities, based on their readiness for professional activity and social skills. Low readiness for the medical professional activity may be represented with various factors: low level of professional knowledge, low motivation for performing professional duties, poor management abilities, insufficient will component and low social skills. Low social skills as inability to interact productively with the others within the medical environment is one of the most important characteristics of a doctor, after his professional knowledge and practical experience. It is impossible to collect the anamnesis correctly without interaction with the patient and his relatives as well as monitor all the treatment process without cooperation. Even more, when talking about the "medical specialist's social skills", not only interaction with the patient is regarded, but cooperation with auxiliary personnel and specialists from other departments, as treatment often requires team work.

Good social skills as a component of high readiness of the specialist for the medical future professional activity and professional interaction may be obtained with qualitative shifts within the physician's **personality**, which result in new, higher levels of personal integrity, transformation of the pre-shaped mindsets, motives, needs and interests, which altogether lead to self-actualization of the person (Hargie, 1994).

It is a rare case when a person enters Medical School with the already well-shaped high social skills as well as readiness for professional interaction, regarding average age of the applicants being still teenagers. Career choice is made presumably under influence of the environment (parents, mass media, etc.), particularly in Ukraine (as well as in most other post-Soviet countries, where motivation for entering the medical schools is originally external, which may further transform into the internal one), so, the students' social skills are unshaped, their readiness for professional activity is low and needs correction, particularly if we consider age of the applicants and all psychological problems related to it. Gradual correction of the readiness for professional interaction and training social skills should be implemented during medical classes, with all tutors participating, as well as by the Dean's offices. This is a complicated process which requires attention of all participants of the Medical School.

GOOD SOCIAL SKILLS OF A PHYSICIAN: WHAT ARE THEY?

Both good social skills and medical specialist's readiness for professional interaction represent an important factor which may provide for better treatment outcomes. Effective professional performance requires not only medical qualification with experience from the physician, but a set of personal characteristics which will provide for conscious and responsible attitude to medical duties, humane relations with the patients, and social skills, which predispose for productive interaction with patients and other doctors.

The multicomponent readiness for professional interaction of the physician includes such constituents as possessing the required knowledge, abilities and skills as well as the physician's ability to apply them appropriately. Here it is possible to speak about interaction with the patients, their relatives and other medical services within the medical environment. Within application of the professional duties we would like to distinguish a separate group of social skills- an ability of productive interaction with the patient, establishing interpersonal relations with him, as this is the group which mainly predisposes for success of the treatment, being an inseparable component of the treatment process.

Interpersonal relations stipulate for any interaction style a person may choose: competition, adjustment, avoiding, cooperation; and its effectiveness: effective or ineffective interaction (Heider 2013, Orban Lembrik 2010). The style choice and performance of a person generally depend on life circumstances, feelings and emotions of a person.

Accepted as a standard, "good", trusting relation between a physician and a patient should be established, with both sides interested in them, though, in some cases the patients, termed by some authors as "conflicting" ones, consciously or subconsciously, ruin such cooperation. In this case, the physician should try to resolve the conflict and cooperate with the patient, and his ability of establishing contact directly depends on his social skills (Todd 1993).

INTERACTION "DOCTOR - PATIENT": PROS AND CONS

Constructive interaction (cooperation), according to K. Thomas (Thomas 1992) and M. Deutch with P. Coleman (Coleman, 2000), provides for the actions which lead to common successful activity of both sides, characterized by such parameters as common aim, motivation of all participants and structuring the process into separate functions; structure, specialization and management of the process as well as coordination of the person's actions. The scientists regard this interaction as "cooperation", "agreement" and "association" (Salas, 2004). In case of competition, the participants act to destroy common activity results, this type of interaction may be called "competition", "conflict", "opposition" or "dissociation». So, we can define constructive interaction between a physician and a patient as that one in which both sides of the process aim to reach the common goal – curing the patient, no matter what methods are used.

Having analyzed the most commonly encountered types of the physician-patient interaction, we would stop at R. Veatch classification with engineering (called technical in post-Soviet countries), priestly (called sacred in post-Soviet countries), collegial and contractual interaction models (Veatch 1981). In the engineering model, the patient is regarded by the physician as a broken mechanism which needs mending, and within the model each side performs the duties, stipulated by the code (Hippocratic Oath, ethical regulations, etc.). This model doesn't count for individual peculiarities, emotions, being a technical one, regulated by protocols. The priestly model is based on the physician's authority, while a patient perceives a physician as the God. The paternalism of the system denies moral principles of the well-balanced ethical system. From the psychological view, this interaction corresponds to the "adult-child" interaction model, where a patient is a "child" and completely denies his responsibility for interaction outcomes, but delegates it to the physician. Here a conflict may appear, because if medical environment accepts the certain treatment standard (induced abortion in case of possible severe retardation of a child, for example, after the pregnant woman has caught the rubella), but the society supports opposite view, then a physician himself must make the decision. The contractual model is based on the "contract" accepted by both sides, with established rights and duties of them. The collegial type is similar to the contractual, but with the emphasis on equal rights and duties of both sides.

Another classification of Ezekiel Emanuel and Linda Emanuel establishes 4 interaction models: Paternal (corresponding to the priestly), Informative (which corresponds to the technical), Interpretative (which may correspond to the contractual) and Deliberate (according to which, both physician and patient interact as two equal participants, but it is the physician's duty to follow all the patient's needs and guide him in treatment) (Emanuel 1992).

Talking about the prevailing "doctor-patient" interaction models in Ukraine and other post-Soviet countries, it is important to trace the following tendency: the paternalistic or priest model prevailed before 1991 and even after 1991, stipulated by the Soviet regimen peculiarities, bureaucracy and strong hierarchy of medical personnel. After 1991, when the country gained independence, we observed changes within the healthcare system which corresponded to changes in the population mind. The newly accepted model of the physician-patient interaction was represented with a mix of the Technical (or informative) and the Interpretative (Contractual) models, when the patient was regarded by the physician as an object of treatment from the medical point, or as a client from the business point. Nowadays, as the healthcare reforms are going on, the Collegial or Deliberate model of interaction is being introduced, confirmed by regulations and educational ethical policy, supported in Ukraine by the Government since 2014, when the new team of Ministry of Healthcare started implementing reforms.

Within the Collegial or Deliberate interaction style one of the most important issues is productive interaction, which, up to the author's mind, is represented with the ability to solve conflicts. We would define social skills of the physician as his abilities of productive, conflictless interaction with the patient aimed at diagnosing the disease, treatment of the patient and his subsequent recovery, with a common linking factor of the treatment process (Lymar 2013). A conflict as a situation in which two interacting sides express different tendencies may quite commonly arise in the treatment process, which evidences about live dynamic pattern of the interaction, but it is important to emphasize that the productive development of the conflict, with both sides coming to the agreement, is the only beneficial one. The physician's social skills define his ability of productive communication.

This is why while shaping social skills in future physicians, emphasis should be made on their preparation for productive interaction. Conflicts during interaction of physicians and patients are common, but it is only constructive conflict resolution which provides for successful treatment process.

Gresham F. M defined basic qualities representing social skills, which we divided into two groups: empathy, social sensitivity, emotional sustainance and altruism; while the second group is represented with communicability, independence, professional knowledge and skills, and the self-control skills (Gresham 2008). R. Liberman stated high role of intellect, altruism, high professional motivation, cooperation skills and high self-regulation which may provide for productive social interaction of physicians, psychiatrists particularly (Liberman 1989).

It is possible to classify all professionally valuable social skill qualities of physicians into 4 groups: moral values (dignity, humanity, responsibility); will component (patience, self-control, ability to complete the goals); quick cognition, including attention and operation memory; and personal qualities (adequacy of self-assessment, objectivity, social perception, flexibility).

So, as we have established, good social skills and high level of the professional interaction readiness predispose for a successful doctor's performance. The psychological components of social skills are represented with the existing mindset of the physician (pre-operation stage) and the physician's alerted attention; his readiness to cooperate and readiness to manage the situation. Medical personnel social skills were studied by E. Topol (Topol 2015), L. Lymar (L. Lymar 2018), Szasz T. S. (Szasz 1956); as well as the issue of medical personnel readiness for certain aspects of professional interaction, including productive interaction.

STRUCTURE OF A PHYSICIAN'S SOCIAL SKILLS

Nowadays, two basic approaches to the social skills and their expression exist: the personal and functional one. The physician's social skills which characterize him as individuality should be regarded within the personal approach, as only personal characteristics predispose for successful productive interaction and high treatment efficiency. Up to the author's view, the physician's social skills, including his skills of preventing interpersonal conflicts with patients, if they arise, may be defined as an individual complex which is predetermined by knowledge, skills, abilities, motives and personal qualities of a person (character traits, abilities, high emotional and will performance), aimed at productive treatment outcome. This means that the physician's social skills, which defined his abilities of productive interaction, are stipulated for his will to interact productively and solve hard situations optimally, if they arise, using motivation, communication, emotional and other resources.

After having analyzed the literature sources and due to the personal experience of tutorship in the Medical School in Ukraine, the author has established two basic components of the physician's social skills: personal and instrumental, including motivation, emotions, and communication, cognition and management components. Personal component includes motivation, emotions and communication, which reflect structure of personality of the physician, his temperament, affiliation, memory, thinking, imagination and many other peculiarities of "self-image" of the specialist. Instrumental component is represented with the management and cognition constituents. This is the structure characteristic for both already practicing medical specialists and medical students, who have been working at it since their first year at Medical School. The structure of the physician's social skills is represented in Table 1.

Motivation (or motivation with values) is represented with determination of the physician to interact constructively with the patient, when even if the conflict arises, he will try to resolve it constructively. The physician should remember that the patient's self-regulation and interaction skills may be affected by his morbid condition, so basic responsibility for productive interaction belongs to the physician. Usually, interpersonal conflicts are caused by unresolved intrapersonal conflicts of the physician, and this is why the physician usually requires for support of a psychologist or a counselor. Unfortunately, it hasn't become a tradition in Ukrainian state clinics to employ a psychologist to support medical personnel, while private clinics in Ukraine pay considerable attention to the issue of personal growth of their staff.

Table 1.1. Structure of the physician's social skills

Social skills of a physician	
Personal component	**Instrumental Component**
Motivation and values component • Complex of the "physician-patient" professional interaction motives, aimed at constructive interaction, particularly under "hard" conflict circumstances; transformation of each situation into the productive interaction in order to achieve optimum treatment results. • Values of the physician, important for interaction with the patient. These values should correspond to general social values and must reflect values of the existing NHS system.	*Cognition component* • Complex of knowledge on the factors of productive interaction with the patient; causes of the "physician-patient" conflicts and methods of their productive resolution. • Knowledge of peculiarities of productive interaction with patients. • Knowledge of psychological readiness for productive communication, its components, particularly the "physician-patient" interaction, its components and social conditions of development.
Emotional component • Empathy, ability for emotional self-management in interaction. • Emotional certainty and emotional flexibility, positive mindset. *Communication component* • Communication tolerance as a non-judgment attitude in communication, tolerance toward the patients, etc.). • Perception of the patient's personality as a partner in treatment process.	*Management component* • Ability of self-analysis. • Ability to choose constructive behavioral strategies in interaction. • Ability to manage stress in professional activity. • Ability of flexible behavioral strategies choice, aimed at the benefit of the patient.

As we have previously defined, all physician's motives which compose the structure of his social skills may be grouped into: pragmatic motives (when the physician "uses" his patients for earning money, making career); social motives (represented with establishing emotional contact with patient, physician's tendency to communicate with the patient to help him); professional motives (the physician is strictly following treatment protocols, with emphasis on quick recovery of the patient); scientific motives (when the patient is regarded as another example of successful treatment); and personal-professional growth motives (represented with physician's will to improve his professional performance, both in the curative and communicative component). Considering these groups from psychological point of view, the prevailing pragmatic, scientific and social motives represent the physician's "ego", as they all are aimed at benefit of the last: with pragmatic motives, this is the financial benefit, with scientific motives this is the benefit from fame and recognition, as well as with the social motives. The motive of personal and professional growth is beneficial for interaction, until it prevails over all other motives, when there is no place for the patient's personality within such interaction.

Though, in each group it is possible to find the motives which would best characterize the physician's social skills: within the professional group it is the physician's will to establish emotional contact with the patient; within the scientific group this is the study of effective communication on the treatment outcome; within the pragmatic group these are new social possibilities established in case of successful treatment (the physician is interested to make communication as productive as possible), within the social group this is communication with patients, the process of communication; within the personal and professional growth this is acquiring new skills and abilities in situations of complicated communication. The highest value for the physician should be mental and physical health of the patient (not an "interesting complicated case"). So we would like to mention the classification of physicians according to their values: 1) a physician with wide range of predominating values; 2) a physician with low professional and moral values expression; 3) a physician with low personal values expression, due to his low spiritual growth level

(Simpson, 1991). Another classification of physicians by life position may partly explain their social abilities:

1. A socially active and initiative physician, a leader of the collective, is socially successful, being respected by the colleagues and patients, choosing the strategies of productive interaction with the others, including the patients;
2. A "good worker", with good professional abilities and upbringing, though socially inert, who chooses neutral position in interaction. Such person wouldn't resolve conflicts positively; as in this case he wouldn't even try to do this. The interaction in this case is managed by the second participant and depends wholly on him.
3. A physician who tends to conformity, led by mindsets and stereotypes, a person without his own mature position, prone to unproductive conflicts, unable to resolve them positively and quite often provoking them by himself;
4. A physician with consumer's position, uninterested in the patient's welfare. The social skills of such person are totally unshaped.

So, predominance of the professional motives, combined with some other points, would make a successful model of productive interaction and good social performance of the specialist. It is combination of high interest in the treatment process, will to care about others, self-actualization through helping others and resolving tasks, establishing new contacts and improving the field a person is working in, which stipulate for optimum interaction strategies of the physician. Shaping this complex of qualities is a task set before the future physician during his medical studies (with preferred supervision by medical teachers and psychological service of Medical School), and further on, during his medical career. The intensity of interaction and "hardness" of interaction situations (those which arise in oncology, in gerontology, in the emergency service) definitely need for continuous psychological support and training the productive interaction. The first step in this may be diagnostics of motivation, with further recommendations on their correction.

Cognition component of the physician's social skills is represented with the physician's knowledge on the essence, factors and strategies of productive interaction with the patient, standards of social communication, e.g., skills of effective communication. The abilities of effective cooperation in small groups and in large groups as well as the resolving conflicts abilities should be shaped during medical studies in Medical School and during the practice. This includes theoretical knowledge of bases of productive interaction, legislative basis of the "physician - patient" interaction, accepted standards of communication in medical environment, types of interaction, factors of conflict interaction and ways of conflict prevention; peculiarities of interaction with each age group; knowledge of interaction basic strategies and transformation of the communication tactics; as well as practical experience of applying the knowledge, acquired during personal counseling and coaching. The author dwells on that it is the responsibility of a Medical School not only to train medical students to treat the patients, but interact with them productively, according to the standards existing in society, and this training includes both theoretical and personal practical part. During the university study medical students learn many subjects related to productive professional interaction: psychology, deontology, ethics, though they are considered secondary after the clinical ones. Such notions as the "team work" and "school of leaders" have just entered the curriculum of Ukrainian Medical schools, and the subjects of "Deontology" and "Medical ethics" and "Bioethics" have been considered important just for a few years. In fact, the changes are not on paper, but in the mind of physicians, and they definitely need time for getting used to them. The state medical institutions in Ukraine have long neglected ethical and social aspects of interaction within the medical environment, and consequently, didn't consider it necessary to pay attention and spend money on social education of their employees, and this has only recently changed, though the private institutions have paid attention to training in their employees the productive interaction skills, in order to improve quality of service for quite long time.

The cognition component of physician's social skills is closely related to the organizing (management) component. It is represented with various physician's behavior practical abilities and skills of productive interaction.

A physician must understand all processes which occur during his interaction with the patient during his treatment as well as follow his own psycho-emotional conditions and control his own behavior. The physician's management, on the author's view, should include well-developed skills of self-analysis, particularly of the behavior analysis; abilities of the productive interaction strategies choice and their practical application; flexibility of the behavioral strategies choice; ability and experience of stress situations management, etc. All these characteristics are based on combination of theoretical knowledge and abilities, confirmed by experience. Considering emotional qualities of medical students, one must note that the skills of self-analysis and self-control are developed after long training and are usually absent in young medical students. The peculiarity of Ukrainian mentality is that there is no culture of "restraining oneself", when a person does or says what he wants, without any limits. This sometimes leads to disrespectful behavior, particularly of the doctors, who may shout or swear at their patients and be especially rude with them. The habit of controlling one's behavior as well as realizing what one feels and why he feels it, should be developed in medical students during their studies; and it would be better if the special psychological services were responsible for it.

Emotions, or the emotional component of the physician's social skills, is also a valuable issue. Both participants of interaction – the physician and the patient experience certain emotions during their communication, but patient's emotions may be affected by his condition, altered physiological characteristics and stress caused by the disease. The physician should regard this, due to his characteristics such as well developed empathy for the patient as ability to understand and co-feel, so, the basis of emotional component is represented with physician's empathy. Empathy within the structure of a medical professional represents a steady characteristic which directly affects constructive relations between the physician and the patient. Both high and low empathy level development may negatively affect the physician-patient interaction model, as in case of low empathy expression the physician regards the patient just as a biological being with some disordered functions, and such attitude may provoke conflicts; at the same time, high empathy expression may result in extreme preoccupation of the physician with the patient's condition, which may impede with making decisions in hard situations. The average "moderate" empathy expression will provide for productive interaction and prevention of conflicts. Medical students are usually characterized by either too high or too low empathy level: in the "childish" infantile personality structure or the "world's savior" structure empathy level will be too high, while in pragmatic students and teenagers who deny everything it will be too low.

The second basic constituent of the emotional productive interaction component is emotional certainty of the physician which is the quality which characterizes a person during his strenuous, "hard" activity, providing for the successful goal achievement. The difference in emotional expression and response onto the emotional expression of the others is caused by ability of emotional self-control of a person. Emotional certainty or uncertainty may be expressed in the strength and duration of emotions, appropriate to the factor which induces emotional response. When the cause of the response disappears, the emotion should disappear as well, and the person would return to a balanced condition. In case of emotional uncertainty the response is often inappropriate to the stimulus: a person develops mild response onto the strong stimuli and vice versa, while the emotionally certain person reacts onto stimuli appropriately. The emotionally uncertain person will express her reaction even after the stimulant has stopped its action. So, the emotionally uncertain physician will shout at the patient if the last has done something wrongly, even after apologies and explanation. Balch C. M, analyzing the surgeon's psychological peculiarities, notes that psychoemotional conditions are of extreme importance, especially for the surgeons [93].

Communication, or the communicative component of the physician's social skills is the last but not least in the list. According to P. Maguire, about 72% of medical students experience difficulties when they must communicate with patients with time limit of 15 minutes. The physician's tendency to perceive the patient as an equal communication partner and make constructive dialogue with him are represented with his **communicative tolerance** (accepting the patient's individuality and his morbid condition, patience to his behavior, non-judgmental position and ability to "smoothen" unpleasant hard communication). Communicative tolerance of the physician is represented with his attitude to the others, patients in particular, who may express themselves in a way, different from the standard one, which may sometimes border on unacceptable to the physician behavior. It is a necessary characteristic of the physician, as his patience to sometimes provocative patient's behavior provides for the treatment adequacy. The communicative tolerance includes: ability to accept the others as they are, flexibility of perception, ability to hide one's feelings when communicating with non-communicable partners and ability to forgive mistakes or adapt to the habits of the others. The physician-patient interaction includes various situations, when the physician must thoroughly explain to the patient his health condition and treatment peculiarities, and the patient must recall all his symptoms. Here the appropriate communication type choice provides for the interaction success, due to sufficient communication tolerance and communication mindset. The communication mindset is a strong view on a certain aspect of interaction, on the person himself and his communication partners. The behavior of people with negative communication mindset is characterized by loss of limits, expression of his negative emotions and unwillingness to interact with the partner. Negative communication mindset may be represented with hidden violence, expressed violence, grumbling, justified negativism and negative communicative experience. Negative communication mindset deals with inability to understand the other interaction participant and inability to emotionally co-feel with the other participant. The person (or a physician) responds to the partner's behavior according to his experience and mindset.

Practicing physicians often show hidden or expressed violence, justified negativism and grumbling. They manipulate and take up the authority communication type. If a physician masters a wider range of communication skills, he is more prone to productive interaction with his patients. This positively affects interaction with the patients. It is peculiar for the Ukrainians to complain about everything, and highly expressed negativism is another trait of Ukrainians, particularly after all economic and political events which have happened in last years. So, it seems logical that medical students will express high negative communication mindset, and all these characteristics should be monitored and corrected further during their studies and practice.

CORRECTION OF THE MEDICAL STUDENTS' SOCIAL SKILLS

The described above structural components of the future physician's social skills (motivation, cognition, management, emotions and communication) are closely interrelated, and with the sufficient level of development of each component the physician will choose productive strategies of interaction with his patients. Speaking about medical students who enter Medical school with unshaped structure of personality and low personal level of social interaction skills development, it is necessary to emphasize that medical schools must monitor all psychological peculiarities of medical students and correct them. This is possible in a few ways: in Ukraine this refers to educational duties of the Dean's office (the Dean's office personnel must keep to standards of productive interaction, monitor the "problem" from the point of interaction and communication and correct the students' behavior. The department of psychology and deontology teaches specialized courses to medical students. These courses include diagnostics of the social skill structure, teaching medical students on social interaction bases and correcting the required components when necessary. The specialized psychological service of the university, if such exists in the High School, may also contribute to this problem solution. We consider it rational to found the psychological service with each medical university, so that the specialists would test the students' personality structure, define problem components and work to improve the characteristics.

Correction of each medical student's insufficiently shaped social skill component is possible by the following activities, grouped according to the problems:

1. Low motivation (insufficient support of the patient by the physician, physician's dependence on the other's views, acting according to the social expectations, low motivation for professional activity) may be corrected by lectures, group discussion of the physician's characteristics, discussion on the physician's independence and self-esteem; training drills aimed at independence; case studies related to the physician's own position; group discussion or conferences on supporting the patient; training drills for expressing support; cases related to support; group discussion or conferences on medical career motivation; drills for the positive motivation of the physician; cases related to professional motivation;
2. Poor cognition component – poor theoretical knowledge on the essence and factors of productive communication with the patient; insufficient apprehension of professionally important physician's traits which are necessary for preventing conflicts may be corrected by lectures, group discussion or conferences on theoretical bases of productive interaction with the patients; cases for the interaction types, factors and basic methods of preventing conflicts or making conflicts productive; interactive drills for recognizing the interaction type, behavior during interaction with patients and ways of establishing productive communication.
3. Poor management component, the "weak sides" of which may be too high or too low level of self-control in communication. In this case behavioral strategies are unsuccessful, with low assertive strategies engagement or extremely high predominance of the unacceptable strategies choice. The offered methods of correction are lectures, group discussions, or a conference on issue of the physician's self-monitoring importance; testing for detecting one's self-monitoring level; cases for the self-monitoring expression; group discussion on possible behavioral strategies applied in communication, including conflict situations; testing one's preferred communication strategy and correcting it; case studies related to communication with "difficult" patients.

4. Insufficiently or extremely highly expressed empathy for the patients and inability to correct one's emotions under the hard interaction circumstances represent problems with emotional component. The offered methods of correction are lectures or group discussions on the issue of the empathy importance for the physician's profession; testing one's empathy level; cases related to expressing empathy, particularly to elderly and dying patients; lectures, group discussions or conferences on the emotional self-regulation in interaction, particularly under conflict circumstances; case studies related to emotional regulation of medical specialists.
5. Communication component with such problems as unacceptable physician's violence in communication; low communication tolerance expression; negative communication mindset of the medical personnel. The offered methods of correction are: lecture and group discussion on the hidden communication mindset, training drills aimed at positive communication mindset development, problem cases; lecture and group discussion on the communicative tolerance issue, theme cases.

Correction of these characteristics requires not less than 25-30 academic hours for each component, but, of course, the best results could be achieved if the correction takes place throughout all medical studies of the student and his further internship practice.

Conclusion

Social skills of a physician represent his knowledge, abilities and skills of productive interpersonal interaction with the patient, according to standards accepted in society and medical environment, which benefit both sides. Social skills of the physician may be acquired after qualitative shifts within the personality, which result in higher levels of personal integrity and transformation of the pre-shaped mindsets, motives, needs and interests. All this leads to self-actualization of the person. It is a rare case when a person enters Medical School with the already well-shaped social skills, regarding that the applicants are mostly teenagers and they make their career choice presumably under influence of the others. Some national factors may also predispose for immature career choice, which may observed in Ukrainian medical students. So, social skills of a medical student usually need correction.

The analysis of literature sources and personal experience of the author provided for defining the following components of the medical student's social skills and readiness for professional interaction: motivation, cognition, emotions, management and communication. Predominance of professional motives, combined with some scientific and social motives, make up efficient social skills' motivation component. Cognition component of social skills is represented with the physician's knowledge on the essence, factors and strategies of productive interaction with others, e.g., skills of effective communication. Management component of social skills is represented with various physician's behavior practical abilities and skills of productive interaction: well-developed skills of self-analysis, particularly of the behavior analysis; abilities of the productive interaction strategies choice and their practical application; flexibility of the behavioral strategies choice; ability and experience of stress situations management, etc. Emotional component of social skills, represented with the average "moderate" empathy expression, will provide for productive interaction and prevention of conflicts. The communication component of social skills is represented with a physician's tendency to perceive the patient as an equal communication partner and make constructive dialogue with him (accepting the patient's individuality and his morbid condition, patience to his behavior, non-judgmental position, ability to "smoothen" unpleasant hard communication). All these components should be closely monitored in the medical students and corrected throughout their medical studies, before they start their practice with the patients.

REFERENCES

Balch, C. M., Freischlag, J. A. & Shanafelt, T. D. (2009). Stress and burnout among surgeons: understanding and managing the syndrome and avoiding the adverse consequences. *Archives of surgery*, *144*(4), 371-376.

Coleman, P. T. (2000). *Power and Conflict. The Handbook of Conflict Resolution-Theory and Practice*. Deutsch, M. and Coleman, PT.

Emanuel, E. J. & Emanuel, L. L. (1992). Four models of the physician-patient relationship. *JAMA*, *267*(16), 2221-2226.

Gresham, F. M. & Elliott, S. N. (2008). *Social skills improvement system: Rating scales manual*. NCS Pearson.

Hargie, O., Saunders, C. & Dickson, D. (1994). *Social skills in interpersonal communication*. Psychology Press.

Heider, F. (2013). *The psychology of interpersonal relations*. Psychology Press.

Liberman, R. P., DeRisi, W. J. & Mueser, K. T. (1989). *Social skills training for psychiatric patients*. Pergamon Press.

Lymar, L. & Omelchuk, S. (2018). Factors of the medical career choice within the context of ukrainian healthcare reforms. *Wiadomosci lekarskie (Warsaw, Poland: 1960)*, *71*(1 pt 2), 211-216.

Lymar, L. V. (2013). The basic components of the" doctor-patient" constructive interaction. *Middle East J Sci Res*, *13*, 06-11.

Orban-Lembrik, L. E. (2010). "*Psihologiya upravleniya*." (In Ukrainian)

Salas, E., Sims, D. E. & Klein, C. (2004). Cooperation at work. *Encyclopedia of applied psychology*, *1*, 497-505.

Simpson, M., Buckman, R., Stewart, M., Maguire, P., Lipkin, M., Novack, D. & Till, J. (1991). Doctor-patient communication: the Toronto consensus statement. *BMJ: British Medical Journal*, *303*(6814), 1385.

Szasz, T. S. & Hollender, M. H. (1956). The basic models of the doctor-patient relationship. *The Social Medicine Reader*. University of North Carolina, 278-286.

Thomas, K. W. (1992). Conflict and conflict management: Reflections and update. *Journal of organizational behavior*, *13*(3), 265-274.

Todd, A. D. & Fisher, S. (Eds.). (1993). *The social organization of doctor-patient communication*. Greenwood Publishing Group.

Topol, E. J. (2015). *The patient will see you now: the future of medicine is in your hands*, (Vol. 2015364). New York: Basic Books.

Veatch, R. M. (1981). *A theory of medical ethics*. New York: Basic Books.

INDEX

A

abilities and skills, xiii, 129, 130, 132, 140, 146, 147
academic performance, 122
academic success, 34, 122
accreditation, 9, 60
Accreditation council for graduate medical education (ACGME), ix, x, 3, 18, 25, 32, 34, 55, 60, 78
acquisition of knowledge, 109
administrative support, 50, 52
Annual Review of Competence Progression (ARCP), 60
applied psychology, 148
Arab countries, xii, 106, 112
Argentina, 89, 91, 92, 101, 102, 103
Asian countries, 108
assessment, 9, 11, 12, 17, 28, 73, 86
Association of American Medical Colleges (AAMC), viii, x, 3, 18, 24, 32, 33, 50, 54, 55, 60, 78
attitudes, 6, 12, 16, 78, 91, 96, 109, 113, 114, 121, 122
audit, 12, 20, 27
authority(ies), viii, xii, 21, 133, 143, 105

B

behavioral change, 20, 71
behaviors, 64, 77, 99
Brazil, 91, 100
bureaucracy, 134
burnout, 148
business model, 59, 66

C

challenges, vii, viii, xii, 2, 4, 12, 21, 49, 52, 55, 57, 59, 60, 63, 66, 76, 106, 108
code-switching, xii, 106, 108, 111, 113, 114, 121, 122, 123
cognition, xiii, 130, 135, 136, 140, 144, 145, 147
communication, xiii, 59, 60, 112, 130, 138, 140, 142, 143, 144, 145, 146, 147
communication skills, 60, 143
conflict, 60, 132, 133, 134, 136, 137, 140, 145, 146, 148
constructive interaction, 133, 137, 148
contractual model, 133

curricula, vii, viii, ix, x, xi, 2, 3, 4, 16, 19, 20, 23, 25, 28, 29, 32, 35, 60, 67, 71, 75

curriculum, vii, viii, ix, xi, xii, 2, 3, 4, 5, 11, 14, 17, 18, 19, 21, 22, 23, 24, 25, 26, 27, 28, 32, 34, 38, 47, 49, 52, 53, 56, 58, 59, 60, 65, 69, 71, 72, 73, 78, 81, 83, 84, 89, 90, 91, 97, 98, 99, 100, 106, 140

D

data collection, vii, ix, x, xiii, 32, 43, 45, 48, 106, 113, 114

doctor-patient interaction, 130

E

education, viii, x, xii, 2, 3, 4, 5, 7, 10, 18, 19, 20, 23, 24, 25, 26, 27, 28, 29, 32, 33, 45, 46, 48, 51, 52, 54, 55, 56, 57, 60, 62, 64, 65, 67, 69, 71, 75, 76, 77, 79, 80, 83, 84, 98, 100, 105, 107, 109, 110, 112, 124, 140

educational experience, 72
educational institutions, 107
educational policy, 107
educational research, 65
educational system, 108
educators, 4, 22, 69, 73
Egypt, xii, 106
electives, vii, 34, 35, 38, 52
emergency physician, 9
emotional intelligence, 66, 68
emotional reactions, 64
emotions and communication, 136, 144
empathy, xiii, 68, 93, 130, 135, 141, 146, 147
engineering model, 133
English as a foreign language, 106
English language, xii, 5, 105, 106, 107, 108, 110, 120, 123, 124, 125
English language proficiency, 108

Entrustable Professional Activity (EPA), viii, x, 3, 32, 33
ethical commitments, xi, 90, 93, 94

F

faculty development, 26
feelings, 132, 143
foreign language, xii, 106, 107, 110, 112, 122

G

good social skills, xiii, 129, 131, 135

H

health care, 12, 25, 27, 28, 59, 60, 61, 62, 63, 67, 75, 77, 79
higher education, 28, 58, 76, 106

I

idealism, vii, xi, xii, 89, 90, 91, 92, 93, 94, 96, 97, 98, 99, 100, 101
ideals, xi, 89, 91
India, xii, 57, 60, 78, 85, 86, 106, 108
instructional methods, 61, 73
integrity, 62, 116, 131, 146
intelligence, 66, 67, 81
interaction style, 132, 134
internal consistency, 116, 117
internship, 86, 146
interpersonal communication, 148
interpersonal conflict, 136
interpersonal conflicts, 136
interpersonal relations, 93, 132, 148
intervention, 5, 6, 14, 83
intrinsic motivation, 62

K

knowledge, viii, xiii, 2, 4, 6, 10, 11, 12, 14, 16, 19, 20, 23, 25, 26, 38, 40, 59, 64, 65, 66, 69, 71, 74, 91, 107, 109, 114, 129, 130, 132, 135, 136, 137, 140, 141, 145, 146, 147

L

language policy, 109, 122
language proficiency, 108
languages, 107, 108, 109, 110, 111, 114, 118
Latin America, 91, 92, 94, 96
leadership, vii, 21, 57, 58, 59, 60, 61, 62, 63, 64, 65, 66, 67, 68, 69, 70, 71, 72, 73, 74, 75, 76, 77, 78, 79, 80, 81, 82, 83, 84
leadership development, vii, 58, 60, 62, 68, 69, 71, 72, 73, 74, 75, 76, 82, 83
leadership development programs, vii, 58, 60, 62, 73, 75
leadership style, 79
learners, 6, 11, 27, 28, 65, 70, 72, 106, 107, 109, 110, 120
learning, vii, viii, xi, xii, 2, 6, 13, 16, 18, 19, 22, 23, 24, 25, 26, 27, 28, 29, 44, 67, 68, 69, 70, 71, 72, 73, 81, 82, 84, 90, 100, 105, 106, 108, 110, 111, 113, 114, 119, 120, 121, 122, 123
learning activity, 72
learning efficiency, 108
learning environment, 23, 69
learning outcomes, vii, viii, 2, 6, 28
low motivation, 130, 145

M

management, xiii, 12, 41, 57, 58, 59, 60, 65, 66, 71, 78, 83, 84, 130, 133, 136, 137, 140, 144, 145, 147, 148
management and cognition constituents, 136
medical schools, 3, 18, 25, 33, 34, 35, 58, 59, 65, 71, 74, 130, 131, 144
medical students, vii, viii, ix, x, xi, xii, xiii, xiv, 2, 3, 4, 5, 7, 11, 18, 20, 21, 23, 25, 26, 27, 28, 29, 32, 33, 34, 35, 36, 50, 51, 54, 55, 59, 67, 71, 75, 76, 84, 90, 92, 95, 96, 97, 99, 100, 101, 106, 112, 113, 114, 121, 122, 123, 129, 130, 136, 140, 141, 142, 144, 147
medium of instruction, xii, 106, 107, 109, 112, 113, 114, 121, 122, 123
mentor, 37, 38, 39, 45, 47, 53, 70, 82
mentoring, 70, 71, 82
mentorship, 19, 50, 52
meta-analysis, 6, 38, 41, 51, 54
methodology, 51, 50, 52, 61, 68, 69, 73, 113
model(s), 6, 23, 28, 55, 62, 63, 64, 65, 66, 67, 69, 72, 74, 80, 81, 84, 133, 134, 139, 141, 148
motivation, xiii, 62, 63, 79, 130, 131, 133, 135, 136, 139, 144, 145, 147
multicomponent readiness, 132

N

National Health Service (NHS), 67, 76, 78, 81, 137
nursing, 5, 7, 10, 11, 29, 113

O

organizational behavior, 79, 148
organizational development, 59

P

paternalistic or priest model, 134
personal qualities, 67, 135, 136
personality, 131, 136, 137, 138, 142, 144, 146
physician, vii, viii, x, xi, xiii, 3, 7, 12, 25, 28, 32, 33, 35, 45, 48, 49, 55, 56, 58, 60, 61, 65, 66, 73, 74, 75, 77, 80, 81, 90, 93, 94, 98, 100, 129, 130, 131, 132, 133, 134, 135, 136, 137, 138, 139, 140, 141, 142, 143, 144, 145, 146, 147, 148
physician-leaders, vii, 58, 60, 66, 77, 80
principles, 12, 16, 24, 65, 66, 71, 84, 91, 94, 97, 133

Q

quality improvement, vii, viii, 2, 3, 4, 5, 7, 18, 22, 23, 24, 25, 26, 27, 28, 29, 59, 78
quality improvement training and education, 2
quality of service, 140
quantitative research, 113

R

research and scholarly experience, 32
research rotation elective, vii, 32, 35, 47, 48, 51, 52

S

Saudi Arabia, vi, vii, xii, 105, 106, 108, 109, 112, 113, 114, 115, 122, 123, 124, 125
Saudi learners, 106
social skill qualities, 135
social skills, viii, xiii, 129, 130, 131, 132, 134, 135, 136, 137, 138, 139, 140, 141, 142, 144, 147
society, xii, xiii, 90, 91, 93, 95, 98, 110, 129, 133, 140, 146
South Africa, xii, 3, 7, 9, 20, 24, 106
structure, viii, xiii, 2, 13, 18, 21, 22, 36, 43, 49, 50, 67, 92, 129, 130, 133, 136, 138, 141, 144
sub-Saharan Africa, 3
Sudan, xii, 106
summer research, vii, 32, 34, 35, 44, 45, 48, 51, 52, 53

T

technical, xii, 66, 73, 90, 98, 133, 134
techniques, vii, viii, 2, 23, 72
trainees, viii, x, 4, 5, 7, 19, 23, 25, 26, 32, 35, 52, 56
training, vii, viii, 2, 4, 5, 13, 16, 18, 19, 20, 21, 23, 24, 25, 28, 29, 33, 34, 35, 36, 37, 46, 47, 54, 57, 59, 60, 67, 68, 70, 71, 72, 74, 75, 76, 77, 78, 81, 82, 83, 94, 131, 139, 140, 141, 145, 146
training programs, 24, 35

U

unacceptable physician's violence, 146
undergraduate medical students, 2
United States (USA), xii, 7, 9, 10, 11, 12, 13, 14, 15, 18, 29, 34, 35, 54, 56, 106

W

Washington, 24, 76, 77, 78

Related Nova Publications

CULTURES OF THE WORLD: PAST, PRESENT AND FUTURE

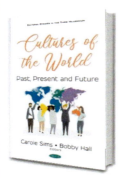

EDITORS: Carole Sims and Bobby Hall

SERIES: Cultural Studies in the Third Millennium

BOOK DESCRIPTION: The opening chapter delves into the cultural roots and historical backgrounds of Chinese parents, giving insight into their behaviour, the effects of this behaviour on the teachers, cultural clashes caused in Australia, and the influences of the parent-teacher interactions in the schools, the local community and also the culture of Australia.

SOFTCOVER ISBN: 978-1-53615-528-0
RETAIL PRICE: $82

SELECTED TOPICS IN CULTURAL STUDIES

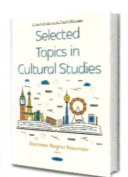

EDITOR: Joannes Ragna Naumov

SERIES: Cultural Studies in the Third Millennium

BOOK DESCRIPTION: *Selected Topics in Cultural Studies* begins by discussing how cultural content can be exploited for designing alternate reality experiences.

SOFTCOVER ISBN: 978-1-53614-735-3
RETAIL PRICE: $82

To see complete list of Nova publications, please visit our website at www.novapublishers.com